Clinical Applications of the Auditory Brainstem Response

A Singular Audiology Textbook
Jeffrey L. Danhauer, Ph.D.
Audiology Editor

Clinical Applications of the Auditory Brainstem Response

Linda J. Hood, Ph.D.

Kresge Hearing Research Laboratory of the South
Department of Otorhinolaryngology
Louisiana State University Medical Center
New Orleans, Louisiana

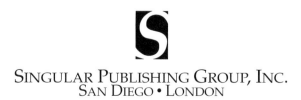

SINGULAR PUBLISHING GROUP, INC.
SAN DIEGO • LONDON

Singular Publishing Group, Inc.
401 West A Street, Suite 325
San Diego, California 92101-7904

Singular Publishing Ltd.
19 Compton Terrace
London N1 2UN, UK

Singular Publishing Group, Inc., publishes textbooks, clinical manuals, clinical reference books, journals, videos, and multimedia materials on speech-language pathology, audiology, otorhinolaryngology, special education, early childhood, aging, occupational therapy, physical therapy, rehabilitation, counseling, mental health and voice. For your convenience, our entire catalog can be accessed on our webside at *http://www.singpub.com.* Our mission to provide you with materials to meet the daily challenges of the ever-changing health care/educational environment will remain on course if we are in touch with you. In that spirit, we welcome your feedback on our products. Please telephone (**1-800-521-8545**), fax (**1-800-774-8398**), or e-mail (*singpub@mail.cerfnet.com*) your comments and requests to us.

Typeset in 11/13 Palatino Light by Thompson Type
Printed in the United States of America by Bang Printing

Library of Congress Cataloging-in-Publication Data
Hood, Linda J.
    Clinical applications of the auditory brainstem response / by Linda J. Hood.
    Linda J. Hood.
        p.   cm.
    Includes bibliographical references and indexes.
    ISBN 1-56593-200-5 (soft : alk. paper)
    1. Auditory evoked response.   I. Title.
[DNLM: 1. Evoked Potentials, Auditory, Brain Stem—physiology.
2. Audiometry, Evoked Response.   WV 270H776c   1988]
RF294.5.E87.H663   1998
617.8'07547—dc21
DNLM/DLC
for Library of Congress   98-27479
                                                            CIP

Contents

PART III.   CASE STUDIES AND REPORT WRITING

Series Foreword

This is the second volume of a series planned as a comprehensive source for audiologists and other clinicians engaged in clinical studies of the neural activity of the central auditory system in response to sound. The series concentrates on the technical and clinical aspects of applying, recording, and interpreting auditory event-related potentials (ERPs) arising from the level of the auditory nerve to the auditory cortex. The first volume, authored by David L. McPherson, covered the late or long-latency ERPs. This, the second of the series, is authored by Linda Hood and focuses on the short-latency or auditory brainstem response (ABR), the application of greatest clinical interest to most audiologists.

Since the late 1960s with the first publications on the electrical potentials generated by the auditory nerve and the brain stem, ABR has assumed a major role in clinical audiology. It rapidly proved to be the method of choice for estimating hearing sensitivity in infants and children and adults otherwise unable to respond to conventional behavioral tests. At the same time, ABR generated considerable interest as a neurological test for a range of conditions affecting the auditory neural pathways. ABR then, developed both as an audiological and a neurological test—a fact not always appreciated. This dual clinical application has important implications for how ABR recordings are obtained and interpreted. The audiologist must not only recognize and understand the effects of hearing loss on the ABR but also, how various neurological conditions can influence proper interpretation. Although the importance of ABR in the diagnosis of some neurological conditions, eighth nerve tumor as an example, has diminished in favor of radiologic studies, ABR continues to have a place in the differential diagnosis of diffuse pathology not readily identifiable by conventional radiology. Hood does an admirable job covering both the neurological and audiological clinical application of ABR. Readers should find the wealth of case studies included of special value.

The major clinical role of ABR continues to be as an objective means for identifying hearing loss in newborns. ABR has recently assumed an even more prominent role as a result of the boost for universal hearing screening from the NIH Consensus Statement on Early Identification of Hearing Impairment in Infants and Young Children recommendation that all children be screened for hearing impairment within the first 3 months of life. Increasingly, ABR is being used as either an operator controlled or automated screening test, as the second stage of a two-stage process involving evoked otoacoustic emissions, or as the definitive diagnostic follow-up test.

This volume is written for both the beginning and the experienced clinician. Hood provides the operational framework for the clinician to select, apply, and interpret ABR protocols covering a wide range of audiological and neurological conditions. The clinical applications and case material Hood incorporates were carefully selected from her wide experience as both a clinician and applied research scientist. Hood's perspective is practical yet grounded in good science. Students entering into their studies of the early evoked potentials should also find this volume of special value because again, Hood incorporates her experience in organizing and preparing class guides for the widely recognized annual course in auditory evoked potential testing offered by the Kresge Hearing Research Laboratory of the South.

Finally, ABR has proven to be one of the most powerful diagnostic tests in the field of audiology. New and expanded uses suggest that it will continue to serve an important role in audiologic practice, especially in the area of pediatric audiology. It is our hope the information contained in this volume will help clinicians develop the clinical skills to take full advantage of the proven and potential power of ABR as an objective measure of the human auditory system.

Laszlo K. Stein, Ph.D.
Series Editor

Foreword

This piece affords me the opportunity to applaud and celebrate a remarkable woman whom I first met in the summer of 1982. As part of a language and brain course at the University of Maryland, I taught a 2-week seminar on the auditory system. There were no more than 10 of us in the room, so to protect the students and myself from inadvertent bias, I asked that all exam and discussion papers be anonymous and identifiable only by some personal number. One particularly shy and quiet woman in the class (trust me, she's now cured!) at first participated very little in our sometimes heated and lively discussions on cerebral asymmetry, laterality, ear dominance, and other obscure but interesting auditory phenomena.

On the 3rd and 4th day I gave a brief exam and asked the students to design what they thought would be an interesting or useful experiment based on our discussion. The anonymous submissions were for the most part acceptable echoes of our discussions with very little new thinking or synthesis. But there was a startling exception. One student, with distinctively legible and orderly handwriting, outlined a set of projects that were outstanding in their synthesis of the problems at hand, referred to literature we had not yet discussed, and in general revealed a unique thoughtfulness and creativity. I found out later she had been trying to get her professors to see the value of her doctoral dissertation ideas and was testing some of them out on me. Her value to our research efforts at Louisiana State University became quite clear to me and I asked her major professors if she could be assigned to our laboratory and be allowed to complete her doctoral dissertation at the Kresge Laboratory in New Orleans. Because we had some cutting-edge computers and state-of-the-art technology at the time, and because they felt she could not execute her ideas smoothly at Maryland because of space and hardware limitations, they very graciously acquiesced.

This was the beginning of an extremely successful collaboration for us; our work together led to her finishing her doctorate, completing a 3-year postdoctoral course, becoming a member of our research faculty, starting a whirlwind national and international lecture schedule, and becoming the fourth president of the American Academy of Audiology in 1992, succeeding Drs. Jerger, Bess, and Northern.

She published important papers on handedness and laterality in the middle latency responses (Hood, L. J., Martin, D. A., & Berlin, C. I., 1990. Auditory evoked potentials differ at 50 milliseconds in right- and left-handed listeners. *Hearing Research, 45*:115–122) and expanded her scope to include papers on electrophysiology in animals and humans and was among the first people in our profession to evaluate auditory function in a gorilla.

The story deserves a digression. Our laboratory had a reputation for being able to evaluate the auditory capacities of newborns in many species; we had one of the first electrocochleography systems in United States in 1967 and were among the first to adopt auditory brainstem response (ABR) technology in the 1970s and teach courses in the techniques to others. (As a matter of fact, this book developed from our continued need for training material for these courses and will be used as the standard text for that purpose.) We had published extensively on hearing in mice and guinea pigs and other animals. At the time (the mid-1980s) the veterinarians at a large metropolitan zoo in the northeastern United States noticed that one of their gorillas was being ostracized and attacked by other gorillas. They thought the victim may have been hearing impaired and was missing subtle semiotic codes. Linda was our most experienced Pathfinder driver (she learned that skill at the Veterans Administration in Washington, DC, with Judy Schafer) and was the natural choice to travel to the zoo and meet with the local otolaryngologist, audiologist, and Nicolet representative to test the anesthetized gorilla. This she did; the gorilla was in fact hearing impaired, but there were no third-party payments for the ABR or hearing aids, and the end of the story is lost in the haze of confidentiality and gorilla-patient rights. I have encouraged Linda to add a section on testing rare and unusual animal species in the next edition.

While continuing to publish important papers and write germinal book chapters prodigiously, she reorganized our ABR courses and helped prepare a class guide that we still follow to this day; her lucid and unthreatening teaching skills are welcomed by visitors to our courses who might otherwise feel intimidated by other, more Socratic, teaching methods. This book, which reflects her own writing and teaching style, will give the reader insight into why we called her "Radar O'Hood" over the years; she seemed to have an uncanny knack of knowing what was missing, what was needed, and what was appropriate to do next. All of her colleagues, including me, continue to benefit enormously from our association with her and applaud this, her first solo author product. I know you too will benefit from her fertile, energetic, and vigorous mentality and I envy you your discovery of Linda's way of looking at applied auditory physiology.

Charles I. Berlin, Ph.D.
Kenneth and Frances Barnes Bullington Professor of Hearing Science
Director, Kresge Hearing Research Laboratory of the South
Professor, Departments of Otolaryngology, Head and Neck Surgery, Physiology, and Communication Disorders
New Orleans, Louisiana

Reference

Hood, L. J., Martin, D. A., & Berlin, C. I. (1990). Auditory evoked potentials differ at 50 milliseconds in right- and left-handed listeners. *Hearing Research, 45,* 115–122.

Acknowledgments

Several individuals have contributed to the development and refinement of the clinical techniques in use in our clinical programs. Under the leadership of Charles I. Berlin, Ph.D., Director of Kresge Hearing Research Laboratory and the Clinical Audiology Program in the Department of Otorhinolaryngology, these individuals include Jill Bordelon, M.C.D., Annette Hurley, M.S., Patti St. John, M.C.D., and Diane Wilensky, M.A. Appreciation also is extended to Melissa Albright, M.A., Lisa Carty, M.A., and David Pillsbury, M.A., for their contributions of information included in the case studies. Special appreciation is extended to Dr. Charles Berlin for his contribution of the Foreword, review of this text, and constant encouragement to his colleagues. Long-term support of the research at Kresge Laboratory leading to the development of many of the techniques discussed in this text has been from the NIH National Institute on Deafness and Other Communication Disorders, Kam's Fund for Hearing Research, and the Louisiana Lions Eye Foundation.

Preface

Auditory evoked potentials provide powerful, objective methods of assessing the neural integrity of the auditory pathways from the eighth cranial nerve to the cortex. Over the years, evoked potential measures within various time periods have been used successfully to (a) evaluate various neural disorders in the auditory pathways and (b) provide objective estimates of hearing sensitivity. This text will focus on *early* latency auditory evoked potentials, specifically the auditory brainstem response (ABR) and its applications in evaluating neural disorders and hearing sensitivity.

The text is divided into three sections. Part I begins with a discussion of the related anatomy and physiology, the generators of eighth nerve and brainstem potentials, and the characteristics of normal ABRs. Measurement techniques are described along with discussions of instrumentation, stimulus parameters, recording parameters, and subject variables that can affect the responses. Part II describes clinical applications of the ABR in neurological evaluation and in estimating hearing sensitivity using frequency-specific and bone-conducted stimuli. Additional discussions relate to auditory neuropathy, pediatric applications of physiological measures, use of the ABR in newborn hearing screening, and application of the ABR in intraoperative monitoring. In Part III, a series of case studies highlighting the principles and techniques covered in the text and sample methods of reporting ABR results are presented. Finally, an appendix contains a series of Laboratory Exercises that review the techniques described in the text.

This practical guide is intended to provide basic information necessary to understand the bases for and applications of the ABR in clinical practice. Sufficient practical information is included to provide the reference information necessary for both performance and interpretation of these measures. This text is intended for practicing audiologists, otolaryngologists, neurologists, and other physicians and professionals in health care settings where auditory evoked potential tests

are either performed or interpreted. This text is also intended to provide intro-
ductory and intermediate material on the ABR for graduate students in audiology
and residents in otolaryngology as well as other disciplines. Further discussion
of many of the principles described here can be found in texts on auditory evoked
potentials, such as those by Hall (1992) and Jacobson (1994), and in the published articles cited in the text.

PART I

The Normal Auditory Brainstem Response

Introduction and Overview

Evoked potentials represent electrical responses of the nervous system to externally presented stimuli. Although the electrical activity from certain areas of the nervous system may be hidden in the larger ongoing electroencephalographic (EEG) activity, it is possible to "see" this activity by averaging neural responses. Through averaging, components unrelated to the electrical events, or evoked potentials, occurring in response to a specific stimulus are reduced. The auditory brainstem response, when recorded from the external surface of the scalp, is relatively small in amplitude. Understanding the sources involved in its generation, the techniques necessary to elicit clear responses, and the factors that enter into accurate interpretation contributes to its clinical utility.

The auditory brainstem response is most commonly abbreviated ABR, but also is referred to as the BAER (brainstem auditory evoked response), BAEP (brainstem auditory evoked potential), BER (brainstem evoked response), etc. The ABR represents electrical activity generated by the eighth cranial (vestibulocochlear) nerve and neural centers and tracts within the brainstem that are responsive to auditory stimulation. The ABR generally is recorded by placing electrodes on the scalp and stimulating the ear with brief auditory signals such as pulses (clicks) or tonebursts. The series of waveforms acquired over approximately the first 2 to 12 milliseconds (abbreviated *msec* or *ms*) after stimulation is averaged by time-locking the occurrence of the stimulus to the computer digitization of the neural response. The ABR can be recorded in newborns, infants, children, and adults with excellent reliability, providing the clinician with a robust diagnostic tool with both neurological and audiological applications.

1.1. HISTORICAL PERSPECTIVE

Electrical potentials emanating from the surface of the scalp in response to an auditory signal were first recorded in 1939 by Pauline Davis and colleagues (P. Davis, 1939). These responses, initially recorded without the advantage of computer averaging, were generated by the cortex at time intervals of 100 to 200 ms after presentation of an auditory stimulus and were visible because of their relatively high amplitude in comparison to unrelated background physiological noise. These cortical responses, or late auditory potentials, are addressed in another text in this series (McPherson, 1996).

Some years later, lower amplitude responses that preceded the cortical potentials were recorded with the assistance of computer averaging (Geisler, Frishkopf, & Rosenblith, 1958). These earlier responses, known now as the middle latency response (MLR), occur between 10 and 80 ms poststimulus onset and are thought to arise from thalamic and primary cortical projection areas (Kraus & McGee, 1992; Picton, Hillyard, Krausz, & Galambos, 1974).

Cochlear potentials, first recorded in 1930 by Wever and Bray, have been used clinically since the early 1960s (Ruben, Bordley & Lieberman, 1961). Clinical recording of these potentials, known as electrocochleography (ECochG), involves use of an electrode placed at the promontory or in the ear canal at or near the tympanic membrane (Stypulkowski & Staller, 1987). The potentials recorded with ECochG include the cochlear microphonic (CM), summating potential (SP), and eighth nerve action potential (AP).

It was not until the late 1960s that electrical potentials generated by the brainstem were identified in the laboratories of Jewett and his colleagues in the United States and Sohmer and Feinmesser in Israel. Sohmer and Feinmesser (1967), while recording eighth nerve APs via ECochG, observed a series of peaks with amplitudes of less than 1 microvolt (μV) occurring within 6 ms after presentation of an auditory stimulus. They suggested that the peaks following the AP represented either repeated firings of the eighth nerve or activity in auditory pathways of the brainstem. Jewett (1969, 1970) demonstrated that neural responses to auditory stimuli could be recorded from the brainstem pathways of cats. These reports were followed by recordings in humans of a response composed of a series of five to seven peaks occurring within 7 ms of stimulation (Jewett, Romano, & Williston, 1970; Jewett & Williston, 1971). Jewett and colleagues suggested that this activity represented activity in auditory nuclei and tracts of the brainstem. They further assigned a series of Roman numerals (from I to VII) to the peaks, and these designators have been used since that time to identify the various components of the ABR.

One reason for the relatively late discovery of the auditory brainstem potentials is their low amplitude in relation to ongoing EEG activity and the other auditory evoked potentials. It was not until sophisticated computer averaging and amplification of these responses, while minimizing the background noise, could be achieved that it was possible to view the brainstem potentials. Although discovery of the ABR occurred later in history than discovery of many other auditory evoked potentials, a vast literature has accumulated describing clinical neurological and audiological applications of the ABR.

1.2. HOW THE ABR FITS WITH OTHER AUDITORY EVOKED POTENTIALS

Auditory evoked potentials can be divided into two categories: transient, or onset, potentials and sustained potentials. Transient potentials represent a single response that results from presentation of a single stimulus. Neural units generating these responses are onset-sensitive, thus responding to the onset of a stimulus. In contrast, sustained potentials are responses that reflect either repeated or continual stimulation. Examples of transient potentials are the eighth nerve AP seen in ECochG, the ABR, the middle latency response, and cortical potentials such as the N1–P2 (vertex) response, the P300 response, and the mismatch negativity (MMN). Sustained potentials include the cochlear micro-

Table 1-1. Summary of auditory evoked potentials.

Response	Latency (ms)	Recording Site	Generators	Stimulus
Electrocochleography	0.2–4.0	Middle ear at the promontory Ear canal near the tympanic membrane	Cochlea (CM and SP) Eighth nerve (AP)	Pulses
Auditory brainstem response	1.5–10.0	Vertex to earlobe or mastoid	Eighth nerve (AP) Brainstem nuclei and tracts	Pulses Tonebursts
Frequency following response	6–25	Vertex to earlobe or mastoid	Eighth nerve (AP) Brainstem nuclei and tracts	Tones
SN_{10} response	8–12	Vertex to earlobe or mastoid	????	Tonebursts
Middle latency response	10–80	Vertex to earlobe or mastoid	Thalamus, primary auditory cortex	Pulses Tonebursts
40-Hz response	Every 25	Vertex to earlobe or mastoid	????	Pulses Tonebursts
Late potentials (N1–P2, P300, MMN, CNV)	80–500	Vertex to earlobe or mastoid	Primary auditory and association cortex	Pulses Tonebursts Tones Speech

Note. CM = cochlear microphonic; SP = summating potential; AP = action potential; MMN = mismatch negativity; CNV = contingent negative variation.

phonic (CM), which can mimic the frequency of the stimulus, the frequency following response (FFR) emanating from the brainstem, and sustained cortical potentials. The 40-Hz response, a steady state potential occurring in the same time period as the middle latency response, is also sometimes referred to as a sustained potential because of its repetitive nature. These auditory evoked potentials are summarized in Table 1–1.

In general, later potentials have progressively higher amplitudes, ranging from the ABR with an average amplitude of 0.1 to 0.5 μV to the late cortical potentials with amplitudes of about 5 to 10 μV. Figure 1–1 shows the time period and amplitude relationships of the ABR, middle latency response, and cortical responses.

Auditory evoked potentials can also be classified as exogenous or endogenous. Earlier auditory evoked potentials are considered exogenous because their char-

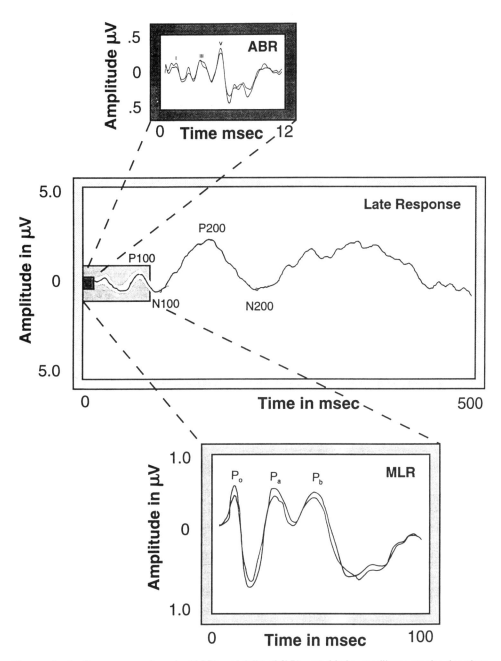

Figure 1-1. Summary of early (ABR), middle (MLR), and late auditory evoked potentials showing relationship in time and amplitude. Large middle figure shows the lower amplitude and shorter time windows of the ABR and MLR, which are magnified in the upper and lower figures. Note differences in time and amplitude among the three figures.

acteristics are generally determined by external stimuli (i.e., an auditory signal such as a click or toneburst). The ABR falls into the category of exogenous potentials. In contrast, later auditory evoked potentials are generally classified as endogenous potentials because they are primarily influenced by internal cognitive processes. An example of an endogenous potential is the P300 response, which is the result of an individual's recognition that a different stimulus has been presented.

1.3. OVERVIEW OF APPLICATIONS OF THE ABR

The ABR has primary clinical application in two areas: (a) identification of neurological abnormalities in the eighth cranial nerve and auditory pathways of the brainstem and (b) estimation of hearing sensitivity based on the presence of a response at various intensity levels.

The ABR has been applied to the evaluation of various neural abnormalities that occur in the auditory pathways of the eighth cranial (vestibulocochlear) nerve and the brainstem. The ABR is most robust in identifying tumors of the eighth nerve greater than 1 centimeter (cm) in diameter, whereas less success has been experienced with diffuse demyelinating diseases such as multiple sclerosis. In these cases, sensitivity is enhanced by combining the ABR with other measures.

Auditory evoked potentials, and the ABR and ECochG in particular, are extremely useful in evaluating the hearing sensitivity of patients who cannot give valid or reliable hearing thresholds using behavioral methods. *Although the ABR is a test of synchronous neural function and is not a test of hearing,* it is possible to use this measure to make inferences about hearing sensitivity based on the presence of responses to stimuli presented at various intensities.

As discussed later, an ABR test protocol for estimating hearing sensitivity should include three components: (a) air-conducted clicks, (b) low-frequency tonebursts, and (c) bone-conducted clicks. Much as different frequency stimuli (from low to high frequency) and different transduction methods (air conduction and bone conduction) are used to estimate hearing sensitivity in clinical behavioral audiometry, similar considerations should be made for evoked potential tests. Click stimuli can be used to evaluate hearing in the higher frequencies, mainly the 2000–4000 Hz range, and low-frequency tonebursts can be used to evaluate sensitivity in the lower frequency range. Bone-conducted clicks will provide information necessary to compare sensitivity to air- versus bone-conducted stimuli. Because of the characteristics of cochlear hearing loss, particularly when it is mild to moderate in degree, *one cannot accurately determine hearing sensitivity on the basis of a stimulus presented at one or two high intensities.* Case examples and further information will be presented to demonstrate both the need for a three-part protocol and the necessity of presenting stimuli both near threshold and at higher intensities.

1.4. SCOPE OF PATIENTS WHO BENEFIT FROM ABR TESTING

There are two primary groups of patients who will benefit from ABR testing: (a) those patients with suspected neural problems and (b) those patients for whom accurate behavioral evaluation of hearing sensitivity is not possible.

Neural disorders fall into several categories and include space-occupying lesions, diffuse lesions, demyelinating conditions, and functional abnormalities of the auditory neural pathways of the eighth nerve and brainstem. Although the ABR varies in its sensitivity to these types of disorders, it is nonetheless a test of choice in patients in whom the clinician suspects a neural abnormality involving the eighth nerve and/or brainstem pathway. The ABR is also useful in monitoring activity during surgical removal of tumors affecting the eighth nerve. This application will be discussed later under the topic of intraoperative monitoring.

During the early years of clinical application of the ABR, much attention was directed toward detection of neural lesions. Now, with advances in radiological techniques and a growing appreciation for the importance of hearing screening of newborns, greater attention is turning to applications of the ABR in estimating hearing sensitivity. The ABR is an appropriate test for any patient of any age who cannot or will not provide reliable behavioral responses on tests of hearing sensitivity. One of the particular advantages of the ABR is the ability to obtain responses in newborn, even premature, infants and for each ear individually. The ABR enjoys wide application in this area.

Although the ABR can yield a valid estimate of hearing sensitivity in patients who have normal neural function, it may not be productive in patients with neurological problems affecting the lower auditory neural pathways. The clinician must keep in mind that the ABR is a test of neural function and that it depends on neural synchrony, that is, the ability of a large number of neurons to fire simultaneously. If a patient has a neural abnormality, such as hydrocephalus or an auditory neuropathy, that affects the ability to obtain the synchronous neural response necessary for the ABR, then the utility of the ABR to estimate hearing sensitivity is obviously compromised.

When using the ABR to estimate hearing sensitivity, the clinician must remember that electrical activity from the auditory nerve and brainstem, recorded as evoked potentials, does not represent conscious hearing. It is critical to clearly communicate the scope and meaning of the ABR test results when reporting results. When using the ABR to estimate hearing sensitivity, one should clearly state that the ABR is not a direct test of hearing and thus cannot represent or describe true conscious, behavioral hearing.

The Normal ABR

2.1. DEFINITION OF THE ABR

The auditory brainstem response (ABR) is a complex response to particular types of external stimuli that represents neural activity generated at several anatomical sites. Accurate recording and interpretation of ABRs require knowledgeable clinicians. Many of the complexities of the ABR are summarized in the annotated definition shown in Table 2–1, which is an updated version of the definition by C. Berlin in an earlier publication by Hood and Berlin (1986).

2.2. THE NORMAL ABR WAVEFORM

A normal ABR waveform is characterized by five to seven vertex-positive peaks that occur in the time period from 1.4 to 8.0 ms after the onset of a stimulus. The "waves" or peaks of the ABR represent sums of neural activity from one or more sources at various discrete points in time.

Responses are usually displayed with positive peaks reflecting activity toward the vertex (vertex-positive), and these peaks are labeled with Roman numerals I through VII. The negative troughs following each positive peak are labeled with Roman numerals and a prime (') symbol, such as Wave I'. An example of a normal ABR acquired from a female adult is shown in Figure 2–1. Ipsilateral and contralateral waveforms obtained from a two-channel recording are shown. The most prominent vertex-positive peaks in the ABR waveform are I, III, and V, and these are labeled in Figure 2–1. The negative peaks I' and V', also labeled in Figure 2–1, are also used in clinical interpretation of response amplitude. The earliest component (Wave I) is only present in the ipsilateral recording.

2.3. NEURAL GENERATORS OF THE ABR

The usefulness of the ABR depends on knowledge of the anatomical origins of its various components. The ascending auditory pathway from the eighth nerve to the cortex is quite complex. An excellent discussion of the neural pathways of the auditory system is presented by Webster (1995). Because incoming stimuli may be processed in parallel, contributions from *different* structures may appear with the *same* latency. Thus, in far-field or surface electrode recordings, individual contributions from specific nuclei or tracts are generally indistinguishable.

Several methods have been used to study the neural generators of the ABR. The information obtained from these studies allows insight into the neural generators, though they cannot provide certain identification of many sources (Arezzo, Legatt, & Vaughan, 1979). The methods used include simultaneous surface recordings of potentials and direct recordings from structures exposed during neurosurgery (e.g., Møller & Jannetta, 1981, 1982), correlation of known pathologies

Table 2-1. Annotated definition of the auditory brainstem response.

Definition	Why
The auditory brainstem response is a representation of the synchronous discharge[1] of onset-sensitive[2] single units[3] of first-[4] through sixth-order neurons[5] of the peripheral and central[6] auditory nervous system, to a click or brief toneburst.[7] It is not a test of conscious hearing[8] but, in conjunction with other procedures, can be used to infer auditory sensitivity.[9] There are many technical errors[10] that can obscure results.	1. Demyelinating diseases, neoplasms, immaturity can desynchronize results. 2. There are other types of neurons such as coincidence detectors, "pausers," "choppers." Acoustic limitations of pulses versus tones (see 7) spread the frequency. 3. The waves themselves do not exist. They are a statistical representation of the sum of single units not in refractory conditions. Note that rate increases make signals louder but decrease synchrony. 4-6. These responses have multiple generator sources and are not "waves in series." Some relevant generator sources are known. The SP and CM can also be used to evaluate cochlear function. 7. Spectral characteristics of pulses restrict the area tested near threshold to 1500–3000 Hz and broaden the area tested at high intensities. Peripheral hearing loss dominates results. 8. There are cases of central deafness with normal ABRs versus cases with normal hearing who have absent ABRs. 9. The test battery concept is critical. The ABR should be used especially with OAEs and middle ear muscle reflexes. Normal sensitivity can be simulated with ultra-audiometric hearing, islands of hearing, etc. 10. Collapsing ear canals, slipped supra-aural earphones, severe conductive and/or mixed hearing loss, artificial "corrections" for hearing loss, use of alternating-polarity stimuli, "incorrect" electrode assignment, failure to use audiological data in patient management, etc.

Note. SP = summating potential; CM = cochlear microphonic; ABR = auditory brainstem response; OAE = otoacoustic emissions.

Source. Adapted from Auditory Evoked Potentials, by L. J. Hood and C. I. Berlin, 1986, Austin, TX: Pro-Ed Publishers.

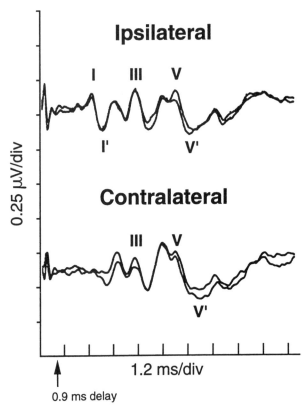

Figure 2-1. Normal ABR waveforms showing replicated ipsilateral (*top*) and contralateral (*bottom*) recordings. Waves I, III, and V are identified. The absolute latencies for the ipsilateral recording are 1.55 ms for Wave I, 3.68 ms for Wave III, and 5.63 ms for Wave V. Waveform includes a 0.9-ms delay between the stimulus and zero point for latency calculation (shown by arrow) due to insert earphones.

with abnormal ABRs, and three-dimensional recording techniques used to identify dipole sources (e.g., Pratt, Bleich, & Martin, 1985; Scherg & von Cramon, 1985). Excellent discussions of the neural generators of the ABR are provided by Møller (1994) and Moore (1987). The following information is summarized from their discussions of the neural generators of the ABR.

The earliest components of evoked potentials recorded from the more lateral portion of the eighth nerve have shorter latencies than potentials recorded from the intracranial portion of the eighth nerve near the brainstem. This suggests that these potentials represent propagated neural activity that is subjected to neural delay. Comparisons of ABRs recorded on the surface with recordings from the intracranial portion of the eighth nerve show that they appear with about the same latencies as Waves I and II of the ABR (Møller, Jannetta, & Sekhar, 1988). Thus, Wave I corresponds to recordings from the distal portion of the eighth nerve and Wave II originates mainly from the proximal portion of the eighth nerve with a possible small contribution from more distal portions of the auditory nerve.

Recordings from the cochlear nucleus correspond with the surface-recorded Wave III, suggesting that Wave III is generated mainly by neurons in the cochlear nucleus, with possible additional contributions from fibers entering the cochlear nucleus. The neural generators of Wave IV are uncertain, although third-order neurons in the superior olivary complex are most likely involved; other contributors may include the cochlear nucleus and the nucleus of the lateral lemniscus. Wave V may be related to activity in the lateral lemniscus and inferior colliculus, but it should be emphasized that peaks IV, V, VI, and VII of the ABR are complex, with more than one anatomical structure contributing to each peak and each structure contributing to more than one peak. The only obligatory synaptic sites in the human brainstem pathway are the cochlear nuclei and the inferior colliculus, and between these pathways there are a series of parallel pathways (Moore, 1987). Some pathways extend from the cochlear nuclei to the inferior colliculi, whereas others are relayed through one or two intervening nuclei in the superior olive or lateral lemniscus.

Although recent studies have provided insight into possible generators of the auditory evoked potentials, it must be remembered that the fact that a surface-recorded component is coincident in time with potentials recorded directly from a neural structure is not sufficient to prove that the far-field component is generated by that structure. This is because far-field potentials depend on a number of factors, including the magnitude of the near-field potential, the internal organization of a nucleus, and the effects of volume conduction. It should be noted that there are some differences between these findings and some early reports regarding generators of the ABR; this may be related, at least in part, to the fact that early studies were completed in animal models rather than in humans.

2.4. CHARACTERISTICS OF A NORMAL ABR

Several parameters can be examined to determine whether or not an ABR is normal. Some characteristics are less dependent on specific recording parameters and subject factors, whereas other characteristics change in predictable ways. A summary of waveform parameters and limits of normal that we use in interpreting ABRs is shown in Table 2–2.

2.4.1 Absolute Latency

The time interval between the stimulus onset and the peak of a waveform is referred to as the *latency* of the response. This latency is, more precisely, the *absolute latency* of a peak because it is related to the onset of the stimulus rather

Table 2-2. ABR values for normal young adult females.

Parameter	Normal Value
Presence of waveform components	Waves I, III, V at slow rates
Response replicability Latency for each component	Within ± 0.1 ms

Absolute latency at 75 dB nHL
    Wave I
    Wave III
    Wave V
	
	1.6 ms ± 0.2 ms
	3.7 ms ± 0.2 ms
	5.6 ms ± 0.2 ms

Interwave latency intervals
    Wave I
    Wave III
    Wave V
	
	2.0 ms ± 0.4 ms
	1.8 ms ± 0.4 ms
	3.8 ms ± 0.4 ms

Latency-intensity function (between 50 and 70 dB nHL) Wave V	 0.3 ms per 10 dB
Stimulus rate increase (from 7.7/s to 57.7/s) Wave V latency shift	 Less than 0.6 to 0.8 ms
Amplitude ratio Wave V/I	 Greater than 1.0
Interaural latency difference Wave V	 Less than 0.4 ms

Note: Values for young males, older females, and older males will differ. nHL-hearing level reference based on average click threshold in a group of normal hearing listeners.

than to other peaks in the response. The unit of measurement of latency is milliseconds, abbreviated as *ms* or *msec.* Latency of ABR waveforms is the most reliable and robust characteristic and provides the core of ABR interpretation.

In normal individuals, the absolute latency of Wave I should occur at approximately 1.6 ms after stimulus onset, Wave III at about 3.7 ms, and Wave V at about 5.6 ms for clicks presented at an intensity level of approximately 75 dB above normal threshold. The limits of the normal latency range encompass either two or three standard deviations from the mean values.

Latency of the ABR is very consistent and repeatable in normal individuals, and peak latencies should replicate within 0.1 ms. Latency is also quite consistent across subjects, which has made latency the most robust parameter in the clinical interpretation of the ABR.

Absolute latency, particularly for Waves III and V, is generally greater in newborns and infants until about 12 to 18 months of age and, as some studies suggest, in adults over 50 to 60 years of age. Latency is also usually shorter, on the average of 0.2 ms, in females than in males (Jerger & Hall, 1980). The influences of age and gender on the ABR are further discussed in the section on patient factors in Chapter 4.

2.4.2 Interwave Latency Intervals

The time between peaks in the ABR is referred to as interwave latency intervals (IWI), interwave latencies (IWL), or interpeak latencies (IPL). In contrast to absolute latencies that refer to the onset of the stimulus, interwave latency intervals use the latencies of earlier peaks in the response as the reference. The interwave latencies used in clinical interpretation of ABR waveforms are those for Waves I to III, Waves III to V, and Waves I to V (Figure 2–2). The interwave intervals for Waves I–III and III–V should approximate 2.0 ms and the Waves I–V interval, about 4.0 ms. Taking into account a standard deviation for absolute latencies of about ±0.2 ms, the normal limits for the I–V interval will be approximately ±0.4 ms. These values are influenced by several factors, including age, gender, and peripheral hearing loss, as discussed in Chapter 4. All of these factors should be considered when interpreting ABR results.

Because Wave I represents activity of the lateral or more distal portions of the eighth nerve, the interwave latency intervals provide information regarding the synchrony and integrity of the auditory pathways from the eighth nerve through the midbrainstem tracts and nuclei and are useful in neurological applications. The Waves I–III interval represents synchronous activity in the eighth nerve and lower brainstem, whereas the III–V interval may reflect activity primarily within the brainstem. The I–V interval is considered a representation of overall activity from the eighth nerve and the nuclei and tracts of the brainstem responsive to auditory stimuli.

It should be emphasized that, unlike some other evoked potentials such as somatosensory potentials that represent conduction time through nerve tracts, the time between peaks of the ABR does *not* reflect conduction time. The peaks of the ABR are formed by multiple responses from various generators and can be used to judge brainstem integrity, but not travel time from any particular nucleus or tract to another.

2.4.3 Interaural Latency Differences

When peripheral hearing loss precludes the use of interpeak intervals due to an unclear or absent Wave I, interaural latency differences (ILDs) between Wave V absolute latencies are sometimes used. Interaural latency differences compare the absolute latencies of Wave V obtained from stimulation of the right versus the left ears at equal intensity levels.

When peripheral hearing sensitivity is similar in each ear, the latency of Wave V should differ by no more than 0.2 to 0.4 ms between the ears. Differences in Wave V latencies between the ears that exceed 0.2 or 0.4 ms are reported to exceed the limits of normal (Clemis & Mitchell, 1977; Rosenhamer, Lindstrom,

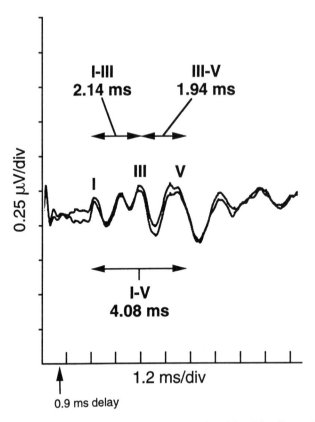

Figure 2–2. Normal ipsilateral ABR waveform showing identification of Waves I–III (2.14 ms), III–V (1.94 ms), and I–V (4.08 ms) interwave intervals. Waveform includes a 0.9-ms delay between the stimulus and zero point for latency calculation (shown by arrow) due to insert earphones.

& Lundborg, 1981; Selters & Brackmann, 1977). Wave V absolute interaural latency differences also have been reported useful in distinguishing patients with tumors from those without tumors (Musiek, Johnson, Gollegly, Josey, & Glasscock, 1989; Thomason, Smyth, & Murdoch, 1993). Caution, however, should be used in interpreting results because false-positive findings may occur in persons with asymmetric hearing losses (Clemis & McGee, 1979).

2.4.4 Latency-Intensity Functions

As the intensity of a stimulus decreases, the latencies of the peaks of the ABR increase and response amplitudes decrease. These latency increases occur slowly for intensities from 90 to 60 dB nHL (the hearing level reference based on average click threshold in a group of normal hearing listeners) and then increase more rapidly at lower intensity levels. A series of ABRs obtained at various intensities is shown in Figure 2–3. When the absolute latencies of Wave V are plotted

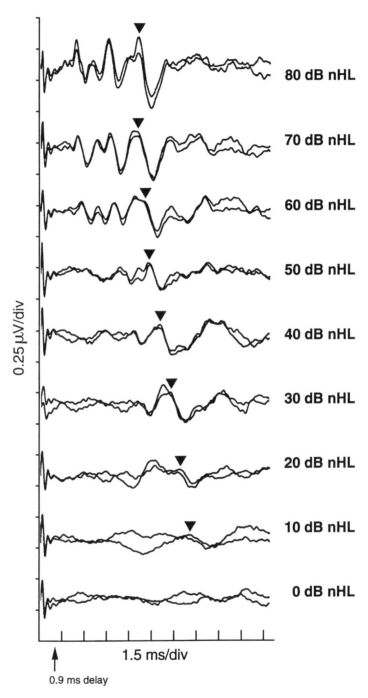

Figure 2-3. Ipsilateral ABR waveforms recorded in an adult to click stimuli decreasing in 10 dB steps. Note that Wave V remains present to 10 dB nHL whereas earlier components gradually disappear with decreasing intensity.

LATENCY-INTENSITY FUNCTION FOR ADULTS

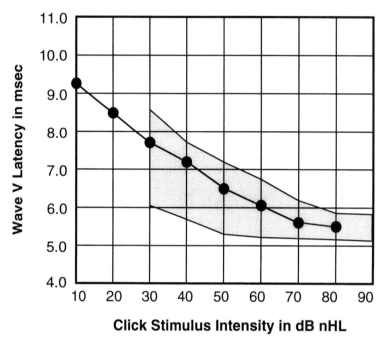

Figure 2-4. Wave V absolute latencies from Figure 2–3 plotted as a function of intensity from 10 to 80 dB nHL.

as a function of intensity, a latency-intensity function is obtained. A latency-intensity function obtained from an adult with normal hearing and no neurological abnormalities is shown in Figure 2–4. An adult latency-intensity function based on normative data from a group of young females and including a range of ±3 standard deviations is shown in Figure 2–5.

Latency-intensity functions differ depending on the nature of a hearing disorder and differ for conductive, cochlear, and retrocochlear lesions (Picton, Woods, Baribeau-Braun, & Healey, 1977). Wave V latency-intensity functions obtained for patients with conductive, cochlear, and retrocochlear losses are presented in Chapter 5 in Figures 5–1, 5–2, and 5–3. Conductive hearing losses are characterized by longer than normal latencies because the actual intensity of the stimulus reaching the inner ear is decreased. In this case the latencies at all intensities are offset from the normal function. Cochlear hearing losses often show a steeper than normal latency-intensity function with longer than normal latencies at low intensities and normal latencies at high intensities.

In cases with auditory nerve and/or brainstem disorders, the latency of Wave V is generally prolonged at all intensities and the Wave V latency-intensity function may be indistinguishable from that obtained with a conductive hearing loss.

LATENCY-INTENSITY FUNCTION FOR ADULTS

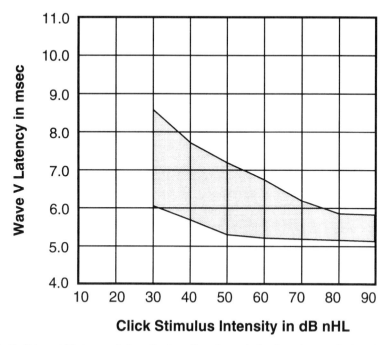

Figure 2-5. Wave V latency-intensity function for adults showing ± 3 standard deviations for latency at intensities from 30 to 90 dB nHL. Based on ABRs obtained in young females (see Table 2-3 for values).

Because both conductive and retrocochlear losses result in a displacement of the Wave V latency-intensity function to the right, it is important to determine the presence of a conductive hearing loss or conductive component in a hearing loss, either audiometrically or with a bone-conduction ABR, when evaluating latency-intensity functions.

Conductive losses can be distinguished from retrocochlear losses by comparing the latencies of earlier peaks of the ABR. In conductive hearing losses, all waves (e.g., Waves I, III, and V) will be offset by equal amounts. In contrast, in retrocochlear lesions, earlier peaks (Waves I and/or III) may be within normal limits or, if there is peripheral hearing loss, delayed by a lesser amount than the later components (Waves III and/or V). This results in prolongation of one or more of the interwave intervals. The potential confusion of conductive and retrocochlear losses emphasizes the importance of having an internally consistent audiological workup available and of obtaining a response with a clearly discernible Wave I to accurately determine the interwave latencies.

Because the ABR is not mature in newborns and shows gradual changes in infants up to 12–18 months of age (Hecox & Galambos, 1974), a different normative latency-intensity function is necessary when plotting test results for infants. A normal infant latency-intensity function is presented in Chapter 7. In general, the latencies of all of the waves are longer than those for adults, but the earlier wave latencies (e.g., Wave I) differ less than later waves (e.g., Wave V).

2.4.5. Rate Changes

Increasing the rate at which stimuli are presented results in latency and amplitude changes in the ABR. High stimulus rates can be employed to evaluate neural synchrony and recovery, and use of higher rates may sensitize testing to subtle neural disorders. When the stimulus rate is increased from about 10 stimuli per second to 100 stimuli per second, Wave V latency increases by approximately 0.5 ms in normal individuals (Don, Allen, & Starr, 1977). Examples of ABRs obtained at various rates are displayed in Figure 2–6. Increases in Wave V latency of more than 0.6 to 0.8 ms from lower to higher rates are considered abnormal.

Latencies of earlier components of the ABR are generally less affected by stimulus rate than later peaks, resulting in an increase in the interwave interval as a function of rate. In addition to latency changes, the amplitude of Wave V tends to remain fairly constant as rate increases, whereas the amplitude of earlier waves decreases. This results in changes in amplitude ratios and emphasizes the importance of considering the rate of presentation when comparing amplitude ratios to normative data.

2.4.6. Amplitude

A normal ABR ranges in amplitude from 0.1 to 1.0 μV. As the stimulus intensity decreases, response amplitude decreases. The lower amplitude earlier peaks (e.g., Waves I and II) may become obscured in the background noise first, with Wave V remaining visible at the lowest intensities.

Amplitude of the ABR is usually measured as peak-to-peak amplitude, such as the amplitude of a positive peak (Wave I or Wave V) to the following negative trough (Wave I' or Wave V'; see Figure 2–7). The higher of the two peaks in the Waves IV–V complex is most often used to calculate peak-to-peak Wave V amplitude. Wave V–V' amplitude is the largest of all of the peaks in ABRs obtained from individuals over 18 months of age and should exceed the amplitude of Wave I–I' (Rosenhamer, Lindstrom, & Lundborg, 1978).

The Wave V/I amplitude ratio is obtained by dividing the peak-to-peak amplitude of Wave V (V to V' or IV–V to V') by the peak-to-peak amplitude of Wave I (I to I'). A reduced Wave V/I amplitude ratio may be diagnostically significant. A study of amplitude ratios in 75 subjects showed that ratios of less than 1.0 seldom occurred in normal or cochlear ears but were present in 44% of retrocochlear

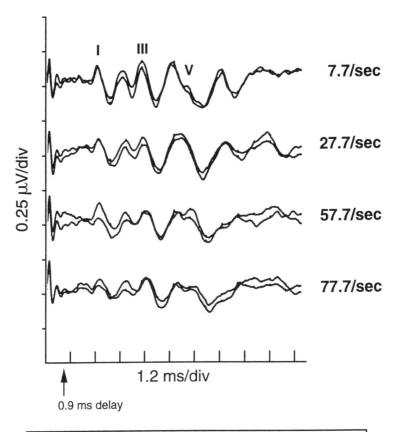

Rate	Wave I	III	V	I-III	III-V	I-V
7.7/s	1.52	3.66	5.89	2.14	2.23	4.37
27.7/s	1.62	3.80	5.89	2.18	2.09	4.27
57.7/s	1.62	3.90	6.11	2.28	2.21	4.49
77.7/s	1.69	3.95	6.30	2.26	2.35	4.61

Figure 2-6. ABRs obtained at rates of 7.7, 27.7, 57.7, and 77.7 clicks per second. Waves decrease in amplitude and later components, in particular, increase in latency as click rate increases. Absolute and interwave latencies for Waves I, III, and V are shown in the table below the waveforms.

ears (Musiek, Kibbe, Rackliffe, & Weider, 1984). Because amplitude is more variable than latency, clinical application tends to be limited and results should be interpreted with caution.

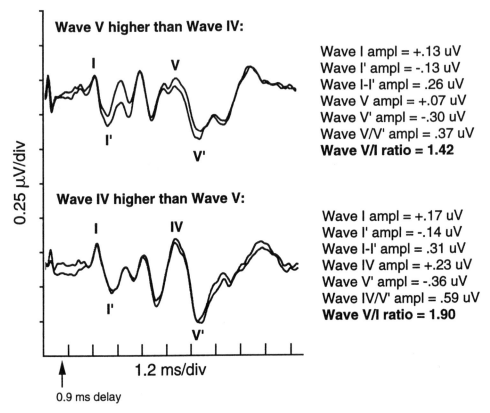

Wave V higher than Wave IV:

Wave I ampl = +.13 uV
Wave I' ampl = -.13 uV
Wave I-I' ampl = .26 uV
Wave V ampl = +.07 uV
Wave V' ampl = -.30 uV
Wave V/V' ampl = .37 uV
Wave V/I ratio = 1.42

Wave IV higher than Wave V:

Wave I ampl = +.17 uV
Wave I' ampl = -.14 uV
Wave I-I' ampl = .31 uV
Wave IV ampl = +.23 uV
Wave V' ampl = -.36 uV
Wave IV/V' ampl = .59 uV
Wave V/I ratio = 1.90

0.25 μV/div

1.2 ms/div

0.9 ms delay

Figure 2-7. ABR amplitude measurements for Waves I–I' and IV–V/V' and determination of the Waves V/I amplitude ratio. Absolute and peak-to-peak amplitudes are measured and then used to calculate the Waves V/I amplitude ratio. The top figure shows an example where Wave V amplitude is higher than Wave IV amplitude. The bottom figure shows an example where Wave IV amplitude is higher than Wave V and is used to calculate the amplitude ratio.

2.4.7. Waveform Morphology and Replicability

Normal ABR recordings obtained at higher intensities (e.g., 75 dB nHL) should contain well-defined peaks and the presence of at least Waves I, III, and V for each ear. Generally, ABRs in individuals with normal hearing contain clearly discernible Waves I through V, although Waves IV and V are sometimes difficult to distinguish. In individuals with significant peripheral hearing loss, the earlier peaks may be reduced in amplitude. Waves VI and VII are not present in all records and currently have no documented diagnostic significance.

Waves IV and V may appear in various configurations (Chiappa, Gladstone, & Young, 1979). They may combine into a single peak, Wave IV may appear on the ascending slope of a higher amplitude Wave V, or Wave V may be on the descending slope of a higher amplitude of Wave IV. These are all variations of normal, though they can present dilemmas in wave identification and determination of latency (Lazor & Melnick, 1984). Contralateral recordings often show greater separation of Waves IV and V and, as discussed later, this can aid in distinguishing the positions of Waves IV and V in the ipsilateral recordings. Variability in morphology underscores the importance of maintaining consistency in wave identification and in providing copies of waveforms with the latencies marked on the waveforms when reporting test results to others.

2.5. NORMATIVE DATA AND ESTABLISHING NORMS

There is no broadly accepted guideline for acquiring normative data for clinical interpretation of ABRs. There is general consistency of data across clinics and laboratories when data are carefully collected using the same test parameters. Thus, it is possible to use published normative data with the proper precautions.

Rather than develop a complete set of norms when beginning to use ABRs or when changing to a new ABR test system, we recommend that clinicians acquire ABRs on 5 to 10 normal subjects (e.g., colleagues) using the test parameters (e.g., intensity, polarity, filter settings) that they plan to use in their practice. Running a few normal subjects is recommended to ensure that a new system is working correctly and, for the new clinician, to obtain some practice with the equipment in the test environment. The ABRs obtained can then be compared to published norms for consistency. Included in Table 2–3 are our norms for young females that can be used as one basis for comparison. *When comparing your normative testing results to published norms, it is important to be sure that the stimulus, recording, and subject parameters are the same for your testing and the results you are using as comparison.*

The primary task when interpreting an ABR is to determine whether the observed deviation from normal is due to a pathologic condition (i.e., neural pathology or hearing loss) or to nonpathologic factors. Many stimulus, recording, and patient factors influence the outcome of ABR measurements. Stimulus intensity, rate, frequency content, and polarity are among the stimulus factors that will affect latency and amplitude characteristics of the response. Recording factors affecting the ABR include filter width and electrode placement. Among the many patient factors that affect ABR outcome are patient age, gender, and peripheral hearing sensitivity. Each of these stimulus, recording, and patient factors, as well as others, is discussed in detail in Chapter 4.

Another issue that must be considered in interpreting ABR latency results using normative data is whether to place the normal range cutoff at two or three standard deviations. Some clinicians use plus or minus two standard deviations from the mean to define the normal range, whereas others use three standard deviations. Determination of the cutoff value is basically a trade-off between the sensitivity and specificity of the ABR in the correct identification of abnormalities.

Table 2–3. Absolute and interwave latency values for the primary components of the ABR (means and one standard deviation for normal females 20–30 years old).

Stimulus Intensity		Absolute Latency (ms)						Interwave Latency (dB)		
		I	II	III	IV	V	VI	I–III	III–V	I–V
90 dB nHL 126 dB pSP	Mean	1.53	2.53	3.58	4.56	5.37	7.09	2.05	1.79	3.84
	SD	.11	.09	.09	.17	.12	.39	.14	.14	.16
	n	14	14	14	14	14	14	14	14	14
80 dB nHL 116 dB pSP	Mean	1.62	2.68	3.68	4.68	5.47	7.29	2.06	1.79	3.85
	SD	.12	.11	.08	.22	.12	.17	.11	.09	.14
	n	14	13	14	11	14	13	14	14	14
70 dB nHL 106 dB pSP	Mean	1.82	2.79	3.85	4.92	5.64	7.31	2.03	1.79	3.82
	SD	.17	.12	.13	.24	.16	.19	.11	.12	.11
	n	14	11	14	11	14	9	14	14	14
60 dB nHL 96 dB pSP	Mean	2.04	2.98	4.06	5.11	5.88	7.34	2.02	1.72	3.75
	SD	.20	.15	.21	.31	.25	.31	.12	.10	.11
	n	9	6	10	9	14	9	8	10	9
50 dB nHL 86 dB pSP	Mean	2.43	3.69	4.60	5.43	6.19	8.24	2.02	1.56	3.64
	SD	.17	.10	.23	.25	.32	.34	.19	.18	.19
	n	4	2	13	5	14	2	4	13	4
40 dB nHL 76 dB pSP	Mean	3.01	4.05	4.94	5.65	6.65	—	1.85	1.71	3.60
	SD	.25	.18	.25	.49	.32	—	.14	.14	.11
	n	4	2	7	5	14	—	4	7	4
30 dB nHL 66 dB pSP	Mean	—	—	5.45	—	7.24	—	—	1.74	—
	SD	—	—	.30	—	.42	—	—	.26	—
	n	—	—	7	—	14	—	—	7	—
20 dB nHL 56 dB pSP	Mean	—	—	5.56	—	7.52	—	—	1.88	—
	SD	—	—	.57	—	.63	—	—	.23	—
	n	—	—	2	—	7	—	—	2	—

Note: Intensity is expressed in nHL (level relative to a group of normal-hearing listeners) and pSP (peak sound pressure). Latency is in milliseconds and n is the number of subjects.

Table 2–4. Examples of two and three standard deviation ranges for absolute latencies of Waves I, III, and V at 70 and 80 dB nHL (based on normative data in Table 2–3).

Wave	Two Standard Deviations	Three Standard Deviations
	70 dB nHL	
I	1.48–2.16	1.31–2.33
III	3.59–4.11	3.46–4.24
V	5.32–5.96	5.16–6.12
	80 dB nHL	
I	1.38–1.86	1.26–1.98
III	3.52–3.84	3.44–3.92
V	5.23–5.71	5.11–5.83

The use of ±2 standard deviations will place more normal patients outside of the normal range than ±3 standard deviations. Conversely, the use of ±3 standard deviations will include more abnormal subjects in the normal range than will the use of ±2 standard deviations (Table 2–4). Thus, it is a matter of whether or not a clinician wishes to "fail" more normal individuals (false positive) in order to correctly identify patients with abnormalities. There is no correct answer in the decision to use normal ranges of two or three standard deviations; rather, it is a matter of clinical philosophy.

To acquire a complete set of norms for ABR testing, the following steps are recommended for establishing normative data for adult ABRs:

1. Determine the test parameters (stimulus and recording factors) that will be used in the clinic.
2. Find studies that have used the same test parameters so that published data can be compared with the newly acquired results.
3. Test the behavioral click threshold for 10 young adults with normal hearing. Their average threshold should be at or near 0 dB nHL on the test system (comparable to 35–36 dB peak sound pressure). If this not the case, then determine how the system is calibrated and intensity is noted.
4. Test approximately 10 males and 10 females (with all subjects either below 40 years or above, depending on the patient population most likely to be seen) using the test parameters that will be used in the practice.
5. Calculate the means and standard deviations for each group of subjects and compare those results to published norms.

If newborns and infants below 12 to 18 months of age are to be evaluated, then acquisition of separate norms or use of published norms will be necessary. Further discussion on establishing norms can be found in Sininger (1992) and in other studies that have generated normative data for clicks (e.g., Gorga, Kaminski, Beauchaine, & Bergman, 1993; Gorga, Reiland, Beauchaine, Worthington, & Jesteadt, 1987; Rowe, 1978; Zimmerman, Morgan, & Dubno, 1987).

Acquisition of the ABR

3.1. GENERAL PRINCIPLES OF EVOKED POTENTIAL MEASUREMENT

Several theoretical principles underlie the measurement of auditory evoked potentials. The auditory brainstem response (ABR) is recorded from the surface of the scalp at a distance from its actual generators and thus is referred to as a far-field potential. Because of its low amplitude in relation to other ongoing electroencephalographic (EEG) activity, attenuation of unrelated activity is necessary. This is achieved through common mode rejection, signal averaging, and time-locking of the stimulus to the recording procedure. These and other theoretical principles are discussed in the following sections.

3.1.1. Evoked Versus Nonevoked Potentials

Electrical potentials in the human nervous system can be recorded both in response to specific external stimuli and in an ongoing manner without the presence of external stimuli. An example of ongoing activity that is not elicited by an external stimulus is the EEG, in which neuroelectric activity of the brain is recorded without the need for any external stimulation. In contrast, evoked potentials are elicited by specific external stimuli and are distinguished from nonevoked potentials because they are caused by specific external, controllable events that are locked in time to the recording of the response. In the case of auditory evoked potentials, these events are auditory stimuli generally presented through earphones. Evoked potentials also can be recorded from the visual and somatosensory systems in response to visual and tactile stimuli, respectively.

3.1.2. Near-Field Versus Far-Field Recording

Near-field and far-field recordings are distinguished by the proximity of the recording electrodes to the actual generators or sources of the neural response of interest. When a potential is recorded from a generator at or near its source, this is referred to as a near-field recording. Near-field electrical activity can be recorded between two electrodes when these electrodes are placed on an axon or with one electrode on an axon and the other electrode on a "ground." Recordings at or near the source of activity are performed in animals and in some instances in humans, such as during surgical removal of eighth nerve tumors or in transtympanic electrocochleography (ECochG).

When electrodes are placed at a distance from the source, such as on the surface of the scalp, this is considered a far-field recording. Because the ABR is a far-field recording, the ABR waveforms represent activity from all generators between and around the recording electrodes. Electrical activity at the surface of the scalp from a number of sources may appear at the same point in time. The nature of far-field recording further underscores the difficulty in discerning the exact generators of many components of the auditory evoked potentials. If the potentials of interest have very low amplitude, such as in the ABR, and far-field recording sites are used, the signal-to-noise ratio is poor, and the desired signal cannot be seen without the use of signal averaging to reduce the amplitude of electrical events unrelated to the response to auditory stimulation.

When performing far-field recordings, the principles related to volume conduction must also be considered because the ABR is a far-field, volume-conducted recording (Jewett & Williston, 1971; Martin & Moore, 1977). Volume conduction is based on the ionic conduction of currents through body fluids. Differences between two points in a volume conductor reflect the algebraic sum of all charges moving through the volume and represent activity from several remote sources. A good analogy is rapid conduction of kinetic energy from a single ball hitting a row of balls. When one ball hits a line of balls, a single ball will rapidly leave the other end of the line. If three balls are propelled to the row, three balls will come off the end almost instantaneously. Similarly, if a few ions are moved sharply into a densely packed area, a similar number of ions will move outward from the remote sites (from discussion by Berlin in Hood & Berlin, 1986).

3.1.3. Neural Synchrony

When recording directly from the source of a potential, the response may be very large and easily seen above the background activity. However, when recording the ABR from the surface of the head, the ongoing, normal background noise associated with the generation of other electrical activity in the body, the low amplitude of the ABR, and the necessity of recording from the far field all contribute to the need to record simultaneously the discharges of many neural units. Simultaneous responses from a large number of neural units, or synchronous neural discharge, is best elicited by an electrical pulse (which sounds like a brief click). A pulse, or click, is characterized by an abrupt or rapid onset and a broad frequency bandwidth, theoretically containing all frequencies. A pulse causes stimulation of a broad portion of the cochlear partition simultaneously, which in turn causes a response from a large number of neurons. The more neurons that discharge within a very brief time, the larger the amplitude of the peaks will be in an ABR recording. Thus, abrupt-onset stimuli are more desirable because slowly changing stimuli may not elicit responses from a sufficiently large number of neurons at one time to see a surface-recorded ABR. This trade-off between neural synchrony and frequency specificity will be discussed further in Chapter 6 in relation to frequency-specific ABR testing.

3.1.4. Signal-to-Noise Ratio Enhancement With Signal Averaging and Time-locking

When recording the early potentials, it is necessary to distinguish a low-amplitude response from higher amplitude background noise. This is accomplished by

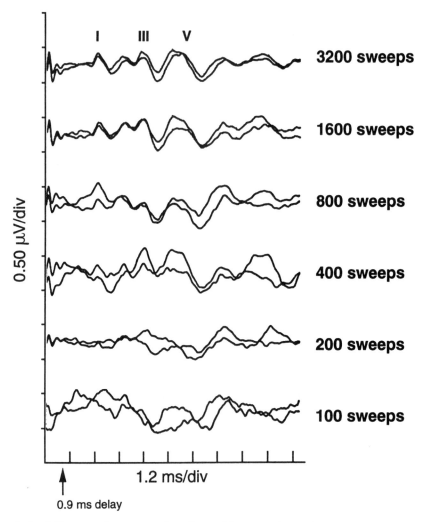

Figure 3-1. ABR recordings as a function of the number of sweeps included in the averaged waveform ranging from 100 sweeps (*bottom tracing*) to 3200 sweeps (*top tracing*). As the number of sweeps increases, the background noise decreases, making the ABR more visible.

averaging a large number of responses together and time-locking the onset of the stimulus with the onset of the computer analysis sweep. Time-locking allows the evoked potential of interest to be summed while the background noise, because of its random nature, averages toward zero and thus is attenuated. The signal, or response to the external auditory event, sums while the background noise decreases. Figure 3–1 shows a series of averaged responses where progressively more sweeps (from 100 to 3200) are averaged together. In this example, the ABR is difficult to distinguish with less than 800 sweeps and becomes easily visible with 1600 sweeps.

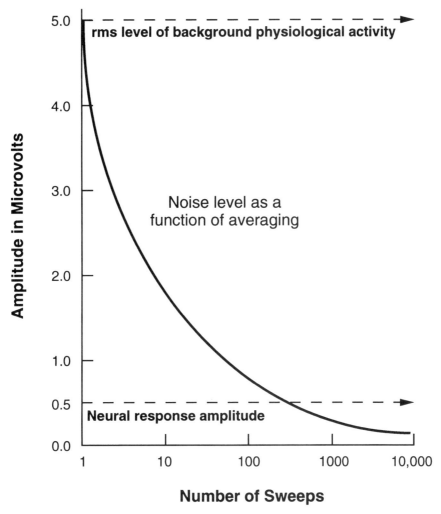

Figure 3–2. The relation of signal-to-noise ratio to the number of sweeps. In this figure, the neural (e.g., ABR) amplitude is 0.5 μV and the level of the background physiological noise is 5.0 μV. The bold line shows the decreasing amplitude of physiological activity as a function of increasing the number of sweeps from 1 to 10,000. rms = root mean square.

The signal-to-noise ratio is a function of the number of sweeps that are averaged together. The physiological response is considerably lower in amplitude than the background noise. Because the background noise is spontaneous and unrelated to the stimulus, its amplitude approaches a zero mean value as a function of the square root of the sample size (sqrt n), as shown in Figure 3–2.

The averaged noise level, assuming that the noise is truly random with respect to the trigger, decreases as a function of 1 over the square root of the number of sweeps. For example, to increase the signal-to-noise ratio by a factor of 10 would require that the number of sweeps be increased from 100 to 10,000. The number of averages necessary to obtain a readable response increases as the amplitude of the ABR decreases. Statistical methods such as F_{SP}, which is discussed in Section 3.4.2, are helpful in making response acquisition more objective.

3.2. GENERAL RECORDING CONSIDERATIONS

3.2.1. Test Environment

Evoked potentials should be acquired in a quiet test environment. A sound-treated room with appropriate acoustic isolation is desirable when recording responses to low-intensity stimuli but may not be necessary when testing is performed using only high-intensity stimuli. Insert earphones are helpful in attenuating external sounds and are highly desirable for testing patients of all ages. Electrical shielding of the environment is another consideration that may reduce interference of electrical artifacts in the ability to obtain clear, readable recordings. Currently available preamplifiers that use common mode rejection (see Section 3.3.6) often reduce the necessity of additional electrical shielding.

3.2.2. Patient Considerations

Recordings of the early evoked potentials are best obtained when the patient is quiet and relaxed in order to avoid artifacts related to muscle responses. Patients are usually placed in a reclining position with good support to the neck and are often encouraged to close their eyes, relax, and sleep during the recording process. An exception to testing with the eyes closed occurs when the patient has spontaneous nystagmus, which produces artifacts related to eye movements. Because spontaneous nystagmus often increases with the eyes closed, instruction of these patients to keep their eyes open and fixed on a nearby object will usually decrease the interference of this muscle activity.

Sedation, such as with choral hydrate, is often used when testing children because they must remain quiet for a long period of time. Any sedative must be prescribed by a physician and should be administered and monitored throughout testing by medical personnel or under direct medical supervision. It should be noted that there is a subset of children whose activity level cannot be reduced with choral hydrate and who may need either other types of sedatives or even general anesthesia. It is usually unnecessary to sedate infants under 4 months of age if they are scheduled for testing during normal sleep periods or soon after feeding.

3.3. INSTRUMENTATION

A wide range of sophisticated computer-based systems is available for clinical recording of evoked potentials. The components common to most of these systems are stimulus generators, electrodes, amplifiers, filters, a signal averager with artifact rejection, response display, response processing, and a means to print test results. A block diagram of equipment used in auditory evoked potential testing is shown in Figure 3–3.

3.3.1. Stimulus Generators

The most effective and widely used stimulus for neurological applications is a pulse or acoustic transient (commonly referred to as a click). This stimulus has an essentially instantaneous onset and is of brief duration (usually 0.1 ms which is the same as 100 microseconds). These pulses are broadband stimuli that are shaped by the frequency response of the earphones and, when transduced through TDH-39 supra-aural earphones, ER-3 insert earphones, or comparable earphones, provide maximal stimulation in the 2000 to 4000 Hz range. Thus, brief pulses reflect activity primarily from more basal portions of the cochlea.

Stimuli should be able to be presented independently to the right and left ears, and most systems allow binaural presentation as well. Stimulus level is adjusted with one or more attenuators. The polarity of the stimulus can be selected as either condensation (positive onset phase), rarefaction (negative onset phase), or alternating (see Section 4.1.3 for a discussion of the effects of stimulus polarity).

When using auditory evoked potentials to estimate hearing sensitivity, it is critical to have equipment capable of generating tonebursts where the frequency, duration, and rise- and fall-time characteristics can be selected.

3.3.2. Transducers

Insert earphones such as the Etymotic Research ER-3 phones (Killion, 1984; Killion, Wilber, & Gudmundsen, 1985) are recommended when acquiring ABRs for several reasons. Separation of the stimulus artifact from the onset of the response through the 0.9-ms delay line in the earphones makes Wave I of the ABR more visible in most instances (Hood & Morehouse, 1985; see Figure 3–4). In addition, these earphones prevent ear canal collapse, increase interaural attenuation, are comfortable for long periods of time (which may assist in reducing patient artifact), and can attenuate surrounding environmental noise more efficiently than other earphone types. Supra-aural earphones such as TDH-39 or their equivalents continue to be used in some centers, though the use of the

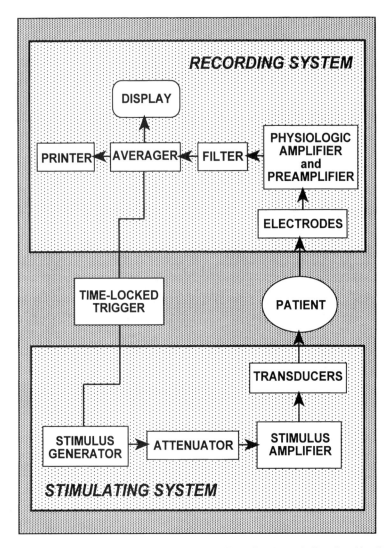

Figure 3-3. ABR instrumentation showing recording (*top*) and stimulus (*bottom*) components. The stimulus generation and recording systems are connected by a time-locked trigger.

"aural dome" type of earphones is discouraged because they tend to produce collapse of ear canals (see Case Study 18).

The absolute latencies of the waves will be delayed by approximately 0.9 ms with the ER-3 insert earphones in comparison to ABRs obtained with supra-aural (e.g., TDH-39) earphones. Thus, when comparing test results recorded from various evoked potential systems, it may be necessary to subtract 0.9 ms from the latency values obtained with ER-3 insert earphones. Some ABR systems can be programmed to automatically subtract the 0.9 ms before displaying the latency

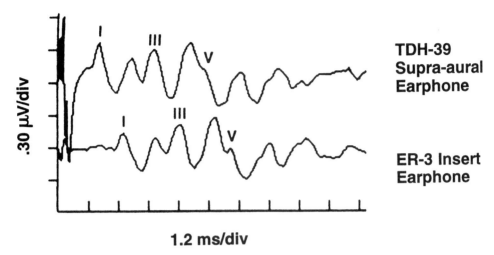

1.2 ms/div

Figure 3–4. ABRs obtained with TDH-39 supra-aural earphones (*top tracing*) and ER-3 insert earphones (*bottom tracing*). There is a 0.9-ms delay in the response obtained and reduced stimulus artifact with the insert earphones.

data. Manufacturer representatives can advise the clinician whether this subtraction is automatically made, or, as an alternative, the clinician can obtain latency data from known normal subjects to determine whether or not the 0.9 ms is included in the latency reading.

Use of insert earphones will affect the amplitude of Wave I of the ABR. Generally, Wave I amplitude will be lower with insert than supra-aural earphones (Hood & Morehouse, 1985; Van Campen, Sammeth, Hall, & Peek, 1992). This may be due to the inclusion of more stimulus artifact in the responses obtained with supra-aural phones, where there is less time separation between the stimulus and the response. The difference in Wave I amplitude will affect the Wave V-to-Wave I amplitude ratio obtained with different types of earphones. Thus, if amplitude ratios are measured, information about the type of earphone used should be provided. Finally, use of insert earphones, by virtue of isolation of the stimulus artifact, may also allow a better view of the cochlear response (e.g., cochlear microphonic and summating potential; see Figure 3–5). Here, ABRs were obtained with rarefaction and condensation clicks. The cochlear response reverses with stimulus polarity changes and disappears when the responses to rarefaction and condensation clicks are added together.

When using auditory evoked potentials to estimate hearing sensitivity, a bone conduction transducer is also necessary. The dynamic range of the bone-conduction oscillator is less than that for air conduction, as is true in pure-tone audiometry (Schwartz, Larson, & DeChicchis, 1985). It may be desirable to have a

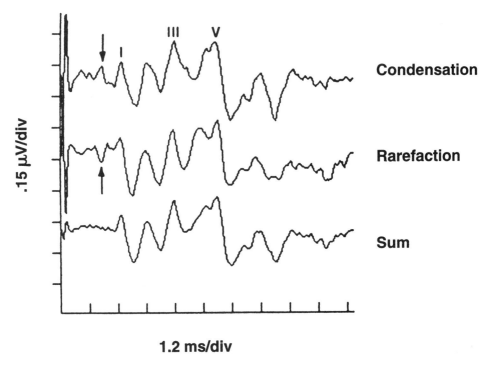

Figure 3-5. Comparison of ABRs obtained with condensation clicks (*top tracing*) and rarefaction clicks (*middle tracing*) with insert earphones. Note the change in the direction of the cochlear response (shown by arrows) with changes in stimulus polarity. When the condensation and rarefaction traces are added together, the cochlear response is canceled (*bottom tracing*).

separate bone-conduction oscillator for the evoked potential system because presentation of high-intensity stimuli over time may affect the integrity of the transducer for low-level threshold testing via pure-tone audiometry.

3.3.3. Trigger

To extract a time-locked waveform from background noise, the computer must "know" when the stimulus occurs and when to begin a recording epoch. A trigger pulse that marks the beginning of the recording epoch can be set to occur in conjunction with the stimulus. Usually the recording epoch begins with the onset of the stimulus and the trigger pulse is coupled to the onset of the stimulus, but certain circumstances may warrant placing the trigger before or even after the stimulus. For example, beginning the recording epoch a few milliseconds before the onset of the stimulus allows recording of a prestimulus period, which may be useful in evaluating noise levels.

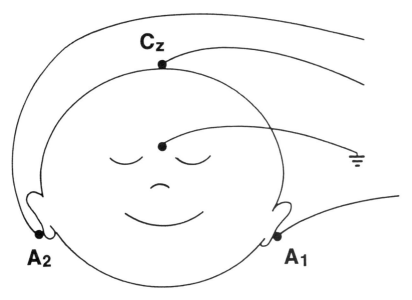

Figure 3-6. Electrode positions used for a two-channel ABR recording.

3.3.4. Electrodes

The ABR is recorded by attaching electrodes to the surface of the scalp. Montages of either three or four electrodes are generally used for recording either one- or two-channel ABRs, respectively (Figure 3–6).

By convention, ABRs generally are plotted in the vertex-positive direction with the vertex upward. This is counter to conventional plotting of many other neuro-electric events, where the vertex is plotted downward.

3.3.4.1. Two-Channel Recordings

Two-channel recordings, using a four-electrode montage, are recommended for neurological applications in order to obtain ipsilateral and contralateral responses. One electrode is positioned at the vertex, which is located at the point equidistant between the right and left ear canals on the coronal plane and equidistant between the nasion and inion on the sagittal plane. Electrodes are also positioned at each of the ears, either on the mastoid or on the lateral or medial surface of the earlobe. The fourth electrode is the ground electrode, which can be placed at any location on the body, but is usually attached to the forehead. In the International 10-20 system (Jasper, 1958), which is the most commonly used system, the vertex electrode position is referred to as C_z, the left ear as A_1, the right ear as A_2, and the forehead as F_{pz}. These electrode positions may also be labeled according to vacuum tube convention, where the vertex electrode is referred to as G_1 and the ear level electrodes as G_2. Although the vertex electrode is sometimes called the "active" electrode and the ear level electrodes "reference" electrodes, these terms and others such as "hot" and "indifferent" can be misleading.

3.3.4.2. One-Channel Recordings

In one-channel (or single-channel) recordings, three electrodes are used, with attachment at the vertex and each ear. Recordings are obtained between the electrodes at the vertex and the ear receiving the acoustic stimulus, with the other ear electrode used as the ground. When the other ear is tested, the ear electrode that acts as the ground is switched. Because electrode connections and/or designation of the recording versus ground electrodes change with stimulus presentation modes, care must be taken to avoid electrode routing errors.

3.3.4.3. Electrode Application and Electrode Impedance

Electrodes are applied by first cleaning the surface of the skin where the electrode is to be placed and then placing conductive electrode gel or paste on the skin and on the electrode. The electrodes should be securely attached with tape. Electrode impedance is measured to determine the impedance between any two electrode sites, though each site generally is compared to the ground electrode. Impedance should be below 5000 ohms for all electrodes, and fairly equal impedance (within about 2000 ohms) for all electrodes is desirable. When circumstances do not allow electrode impedance below 5000 ohms, it is particularly important to try to balance the impedance so that all electrodes have impedances within 2000 ohms of each other. Fairly equal electrode impedance facilitates the efficiency of the common mode rejection system, which serves to minimize background interference. Electrode impedance should be checked after the earphones and patient are positioned for testing and periodically during testing because changes in impedance may affect the quality of the recordings.

3.3.5. Preamplifiers

Preamplifiers are the second stage of the recording system and the attachment point for the electrodes. The preamplifiers are either near the attachment point of the electrodes or connected to the electrodes through an electrode input box and cable. When the preamplifiers are near the point of electrode attachment, some advantage in the signal-to-noise ratio may be obtained because the low-amplitude signals will need to travel less distance. Because of the low amplitude of the ABR (on the order of 0.1 to 1.0 μV), a companion amplifier and a preamplifier may be necessary to provide amplification of the signal by about 100,000 times. Amplification of the neural activity places the response into a range that can be processed by the signal averager.

3.3.6. Common Mode Rejection

Evoked potential recordings of interest are recorded between two electrodes. By using a differential amplifier, the voltages at each of the two electrodes in a pair (e.g., C_z and A_1) are subtracted from each other. Consider, for example, recordings obtained between the vertex (C_z) and left ear (A_1). If the C_z electrode is selected as the vertex-positive-upward electrode, then voltages propagated toward that electrode are slightly different than voltages at the A_1 electrode, which is positioned at the left ear. The electrical activity contains both the desired signal related to the response of the auditory neural pathways to the acoustic stimulus and unrelated electrical noise from the body (e.g., EEG and electrocardiogram) and the environment (e.g., a local radio station).

The unrelated and outside electrical activity is common to both electrodes and has the same value. When the voltages at each of the electrodes (in this example C_z and A_1) are subtracted from each other, electrical activity common to both electrodes is canceled (called common mode rejection) and the remaining voltage is that which actually differs between the two electrodes, ideally the target potential (Figure 3–7). For common mode rejection to work most efficiently, the impedance should be similar at the two electrodes.

3.3.7. Filters

Filtering of the physiological response is another way to remove some of the unwanted electrical activity. Filtering in this case is performed on the biological signal coming from the electrodes. This is distinguished from filtering of the acoustic stimulus, a common practice in other types of auditory testing. A bandpass filter is set in evoked potential testing to remove as much of the background noise and unwanted electrical activity as possible without affecting the frequency range of the evoked potential of interest.

For ABR testing with click stimuli, filter settings of either 100 or 150 Hz on the low-frequency end (high-pass setting) and 3000 Hz on the high-frequency end (low-pass setting) with slopes of either 6 or 12 dB per octave are most commonly used. It is sometimes useful to decrease the high-pass (low-end) filter setting to 30 Hz to emphasize Wave V. When recording the ABR using low-frequency tonebursts such as 500 Hz, filter settings of 30 to 1500 Hz are recommended to emphasize Wave V, the primary component in low-frequency toneburst ABRs. A high-pass setting of 30 Hz is also recommended when testing infants. For ECochG, filter settings of 30 to 3000 Hz are recommended to include the lower frequency summating potential. For later latency auditory evoked potentials, such as the middle latency response or late N_1–P_2 response, filter settings will be in the 1 to 100 Hz range because these potentials are lower in frequency. Thus, knowledge of the frequency characteristics of the evoked potential of interest determines the necessary filter settings.

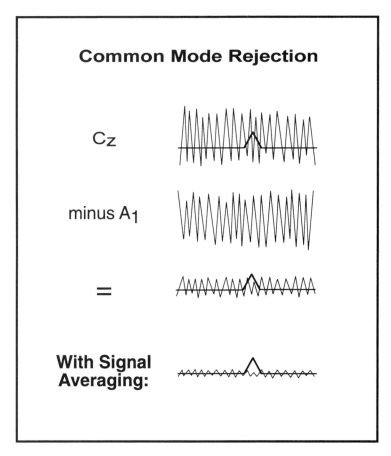

Figure 3-7. Effects of common mode rejection and signal averaging. The response (a single peak) and noise are shown at the vertex electrode (*top figure*). The use of common mode rejection allows subtraction of the response at the ear from the vertex response, resulting in reduced noise. With signal averaging (shown at the bottom), the noise is further reduced so that the desired response can be seen.

In addition to filtering that is completed during data acquisition, post hoc digital filtering can be used to further remove unwanted frequencies from the ABR. Although digital filtering cannot remove all noise, it can be helpful in some situations to improve ability to identify waveforms, particularly the earlier components (Lettrem & Laukli, 1995).

3.3.8. Signal Averager

The signal averager converts the analog electrical activity from the amplifiers (the physiological response) into a series of numerical (digital) values. These digital values are processed by the computer to generate the summed or averaged re-

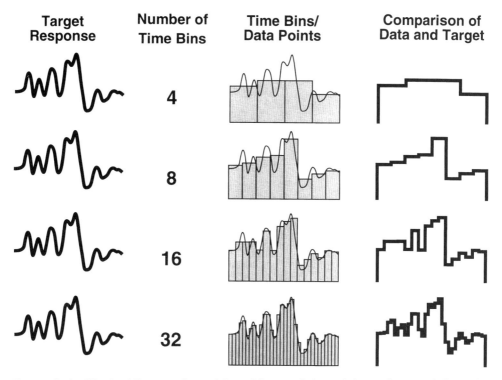

| Target Response | Number of Time Bins | Time Bins/ Data Points | Comparison of Data and Target |

Figure 3-8. Effect of the number of time bins or data points on the resolution of a waveform. In this figure, the ABR is the target response (shown in the left panel), and the number of data points collected varies from 4 to 32. As seen in the right panel, the waveform begins to resolve as the number of data points increases. In practice 256 or 512 data points are generally used to define the ABR.

sponse. The time period in which the response of interest occurs determines the time window set for collection of digital values (about 10 to 15 ms after the stimulus in the case of the ABR to clicks). This time window is broken down into a series of time units, time bins, or data points after the occurrence of the stimulus. Activity that is related to the acoustic stimulus occurs consistently in the same time periods or time bins after each stimulus is presented. Thus, over successive presentations, positive values consistently accumulate in some time bins and negative values in others, resulting in the familiar response waveforms.

The number of time bins or data points contained in a particular time period is related to the digitizing rate of the computer, the resolution of the computer system, and the number of waveforms obtained simultaneously. The resolution may be adjusted according to the frequency range of the desired response and should be sufficiently high to ensure that the details of the response are recorded but with the sampling rate below the Nyquist frequency. Figure 3–8 shows a schematic of the effects of increasing the number of data points. In practice 256 to 512 data points are used to resolve the ABR.

Because the frequency characteristics of the ABR are higher than later cortical potentials, data must be collected in narrower time periods in order to define all of the peaks and valleys of the composite ABR waveform. Data points further apart in time are sufficient for later, lower frequency evoked potentials. The digitizing rate and the resolution of the system must be appropriate for the evoked potential being recorded.

3.3.9. Display of Responses

Visual displays are provided of the waveform as it is either averaged or summed. In addition, some equipment allows the operator to view the ongoing individual sweeps either simultaneously or alternately with the averaged or summed accumulation of the response. Viewing the ongoing activity allows the operator to identify periods of excessive activity such as when the patient moves or external electrical artifacts interfere with the recording. The operator can then decide whether valid data are being collected and can discontinue the run if the recording quality is poor.

3.3.10. Artifact Rejection

When a sweep occurs that contains excessive voltage amplitudes, excessive noise is included in the average, which can decrease the quality of a recording. Most evoked potential systems provide a method where sweeps containing excessive noise can be excluded from the ongoing average. This is known as artifact rejection. The artifact rejection level is set so that sweeps containing voltages well above the voltages of the response of interest are rejected and thus not added into the summed or averaged response. For the ABR, which is in the range of 0.1 to 1.0 μV, a typical artifact rejection level might be 10 μV. This will serve to exclude large electrical responses, such as those related to muscle activity or the environment, while including the response of interest, in this case the ABR. On rare occasions it may be necessary to either increase the rejection level or deactivate the artifact rejection system. When this is done, the operator should watch the ongoing EEG activity carefully and pause the system whenever high electrical or other interfering activity is observed.

3.3.11. Data Analysis and Storage

Most evoked potential systems allow storage of accumulated data on disks. Storage of the original waveforms prior to addition or subtraction is best because additional analyses of the raw data may be desired at a later date. When interpreting data, the utility of recalling waves and adding, subtracting, or overlaying them as well as reanalyzing latency information can be invaluable. The ability to store responses and then recall them at a later time for reanalysis or comparison to subsequent test results strengthens the utility of evoked potential testing.

Hard-copy plots of responses display time on the abscissa (horizontal, or X, axis) and amplitude on the ordinate (vertical, or Y, axis). All waveforms that contribute to the interpretation of the evoked potential test results should be printed and included in the patient's chart as well as sent out with reports.

3.3.12. Calibration

Physical calibration of the stimuli used for evoked potential testing requires considerations beyond those related to pure-tone calibration of audiometers due to the short duration of the pulses or tonebursts. Two methods can be used to express the sound pressure (SP) of the stimuli: peak SP and peak equivalent SP. Peak SP is the intensity of the pulse at the maximal point of pressure and is measured on a sound level meter that has a peak-hold capacity. Sound level meters without the peak-hold capacity are unable to capture the maximum pressure because of the long integration time, which requires longer duration stimuli than those used in early evoked potential recording. Peak equivalent SP is obtained by comparison of a pulse to a pure tone having the same peak amplitude. This is accomplished using an oscilloscope to compare the peaks of the pulse and the pure tone and a sound level meter to read the actual SPs.

Biological references relate the intensity of a pulse or toneburst to the average threshold of a group of normal-hearing young adults (Picton, Woods, Baribeau-Braun, & Healey, 1977). This method yields a hearing level (HL) reference, noted as nHL or HLN, which is similar in principle to the standard HL references used for pure tones. Stapells, Picton, and Smith (1982) reported that the average behavioral threshold in young adults for 100-microsecond pulses presented through TDH-49 earphones at a rate of 10 per second is 36.4 dB peak SP and 29.9 dB peak equivalent SP.

Behavioral thresholds for fast stimulation rates are more sensitive than behavioral thresholds for slow presentation rates. Changes of 4.5 dB for a tenfold increase in rate (Stapells et al., 1982) and 6 dB for an increase from 13 per second to 67 per second (Weber, Seitz, & McCutcheon, 1981) have been reported.

3.4. SPECIALIZED TECHNIQUES IN ABR ACQUISITION

3.4.1. Signal-to-Noise Estimation

Using statistical techniques, it is possible to determine the quality of an ABR recording based on an estimate of the overall noise level in the response. Methods involving signal-to-noise ratio (SNR) estimation during evoked potential averaging are employed in evoked potential testing to assist in determination of the presence of a response in relation to the background noise levels. Studies where various methods of signal-to-noise ratio estimation have been applied to ABR averaging show that the quality of the averaged response can be quantitatively assessed by continuous display of the signal-to-noise ratio and residual noise estimates during the averaging process (e.g., Özdamar & Delgado, 1996). These and other signal-to-noise estimation algorithms are useful in attempting to quantify response characteristics and thus make interpretation of response presence less subjective.

3.4.2. F_{SP} Averaging

A method of signal and noise estimation, referred to as F_{SP}, was developed by Elberling and Don (1984) that uses statistical properties of the response to determine when an acceptable signal-to-noise relationship in the averaged response is reached. F denotes an F ratio and SP a single point in the time window of the response. The F_{SP} method calculates an F ratio that compares the variance of the averaged response (an estimate of the averaged signal and the noise) to the variance of the amplitude of a single point at a given time in each sweep (which is an estimate of the background noise).

When an F ratio of a predetermined level is reached in the accumulation of sweeps, averaging is stopped based on the theory that further accumulation of averages will not significantly improve the F ratio (and thus the signal-to-noise ratio). Generally, larger F ratios are achieved more quickly for high-intensity stimuli in individuals with normal ABRs, so fewer averages are necessary (Don, Elberling, & Waring, 1984). Nearer threshold, and in patients with abnormal ABRs, more sweeps are generally necessary to obtain acceptable F_{SP} values, and sometimes at threshold or in dissynchronous ABRs, an acceptable level is never reached. This method is useful in limiting the number of averages necessary at high intensities where the ABR amplitude is high in relation to the noise level and in determining when further averaging will not improve a response. Use of F_{SP} offers great advantages in decreasing acquisition time at higher intensities, providing an objective method of determining acceptable signal-to-noise relationships in responses, and objectively determining when an appropriate number of averages have been obtained (Don & Elberling, 1996; Sininger, 1993).

3.4.3. Maximum Length Sequences (MLS)

Traditional ABR acquisition techniques allow completion of data acquisition for each sweep prior to the presentation of the next stimulus. Thus, if the time window is set at 10 ms, a maximum stimulus rate of 100 per second would be possible (100 stimuli × 10-ms window = 1000 ms or 1 s). By utilizing specialized stimuli called maximum length sequences (MLS) and a specialized analysis technique (Eysholdt & Schreiner, 1982), it is possible to acquire ABRs using very rapid stimulus presentation rates (Picton, Champagne, & Kellett, 1992; Thornton & Slaven, 1993).

Stimuli are presented in specially constructed pseudorandom binary sequences that allow acquisition of more than one transient response within the same time period. Individual responses also can be obtained from both ears at the same time through presentation of different sequences to each ear (such as in a binaural asynchronous mode). After acquisition, the overlapping responses are then deconvoluted to recapture the ABR into the familiar format. With this technique, monaural ABRs from both ears at several intensity levels can be obtained in one fourth to one third of the time required using traditional averaging techniques. Standard ABRs and MLS ABRs obtained at several intensities are shown in Figure 3–9. Total test time for click stimuli for both ears with the MLS technique was less than 5 min.

The latency of the MLS response is slightly longer than with traditional techniques and the amplitude of the earlier components is often attenuated, whereas threshold estimates are comparable between methods. A number of studies have demonstrated the utility of the MLS method in infants and adults (Lasky, Shi, & Hecox, 1993; Lina-Grande, Collet, & Morgon, 1994; Weber & Roush, 1993). Examples of ABRs obtained with the MLS technique compared to traditional ABRs also are shown in Case Studies 11 and 15.

3.4.4. Automated Identification of Waveforms

Several computer algorithms have been developed to provide rapid identification of peaks in the ABR (e.g., Mason, 1984; Özdamar, Delgado, Eilers, & Urbano, 1994; Pool & Finitzo, 1989). Generally these programs identify the highest amplitudes in latency regions where peaks are expected to occur in a normal ABR. Features that are considered include aspects of the response that expert ABR judges consider, such as similarity with a normal template, reliability of a response, and morphological characteristics (Sanchez, Riquenes, & Perez-Abalo, 1995). Some programs provide initial markings of waveforms that are then confirmed by the clinician, whereas other automated systems depend on algorithms to identify responses without confirmation by the examiner. Each method has advantages and disadvantages, and clinicians should be aware of these and able to confirm efficiency of their use in their particular patient population.

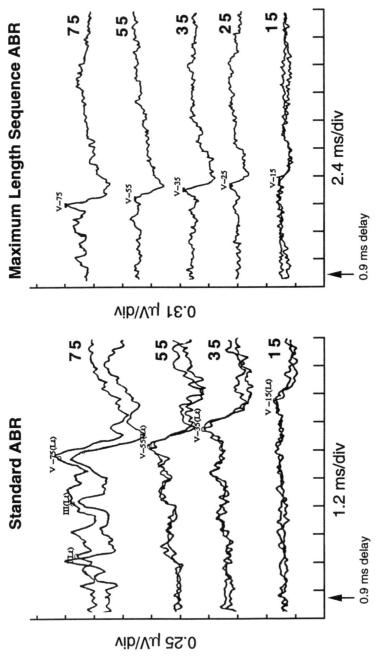

Figure 3–9. Comparison of a standard ABR intensity series, shown at the left, and ABRs obtained using maximum length sequences, shown at the right. Note the differences in the time base.

4

Stimulus, Recording, and Patient Factors Influencing the ABR

A number of stimulus, recording, and patient factors, as listed in Table 4–1, influence the auditory brainstem response (ABR). These factors may affect the latency and/or amplitude of the waveforms. Thus, it is important for the clinician to understand these effects and apply them to both recording and interpretation of ABRs.

4.1. EFFECTS OF STIMULUS FACTORS

Manipulations of test stimuli affect both the latency and the amplitude of the early evoked potentials. An understanding of the effects of these manipulations is necessary to obtain the best possible responses and to correctly interpret test results.

4.1.1. Stimulus Intensity

All waves of the ABR show a systematic increase in latency and decrease in amplitude as stimulus intensity decreases from 70 or 80 dB nHL to the threshold of detectability (Picton et al., 1974; Starr & Achor, 1975). This is illustrated in Figure 2–3. Wave V is most visible at lower intensity levels, whereas the earlier components tend to become indistinguishable at intensities of 25 to 35 dB nHL. Near the threshold of the response, Wave I occurs at approximately 4.0 ms and Wave V at about 8.0 ms in adults. Absolute and interwave latencies for the primary components of the ABR are shown in Table 2–3 for a series of female subjects between 20 and 30 years old.

The Wave V latency shift with changes in intensity is nonlinear, with shifts of approximately 0.2 to 0.3 ms per 10 dB at higher intensities and a steeper slope at lower intensities. Wave V latencies from Figure 2–3 are plotted onto an adult latency-intensity (L-I) function in Figure 2–4. As intensity is reduced from 70 to 30 dB nHL, the latency shift is the greatest for Wave I and least for Wave V

Table 4–1. Summary of stimulus, recording, and patient factors affecting the ABR.

Stimulus Factors	Recording Factors	Patient Factors
Intensity	Electrode montage	Age
Rate	Filter settings	Gender
Polarity	Time window	Medications
Duration/rise time	Number of channels	Attention
Frequency	Number of sweeps	Body temperature
Monaural/binaural		Muscle artifact

(Stockard, Stockard, Westmoreland, & Corfits, 1979). This can result in an inter-wave latency interval that is slightly shorter at lower intensities.

The amplitude of the ABR is rarely greater than 1 μV and no consistent values in amplitude growth as a function of intensity have been reported (Hecox & Galambos, 1974; Jewett & Williston, 1971). This is most likely related to the considerable variation in amplitude within and among subjects. Generally, the amplitude of the Waves IV/V complex is less affected by intensity decreases than earlier components (Pratt & Sohmer, 1976; Terkildsen, Osterhammel, & Huis in't Veld, 1975).

It is important to note that the actual intensity and frequency information reaching the cochlea are dependent on the acoustic properties of the transducer, the volume of the external ear canal, and middle ear transmission characteristics. Current technological advances should facilitate use in the future of (a) a transducer containing a probe microphone to monitor the actual sound pressure level generated in the ear canal and (b) a method to account for intensity differences as a function of ear canal volume. Such advances should be especially useful in neonatal screening and testing of infants and young children.

4.1.2. Stimulus Rate

The rate at which test stimuli are presented affects both the latency and the amplitude of the components of the ABR. In general, at stimulus rates above approximately 30 stimuli per second, the latency of all components of the ABR increases and the amplitude of the earlier components decreases (Don et al., 1977; Fowler & Noffsinger, 1983; Hyde, Stephens, & Thornton, 1976; Paludetti, Maurizi, & Ottaviani, 1983; Pratt & Sohmer, 1976; Terkildsen et al., 1975; van Olphen, Rodenburg, & Verwey, 1979).

Latency does not increase by the same amount for all components. The later waves of the ABR (e.g., Wave V) show a greater latency increase than the earlier waves, which results in a prolongation of the interwave interval of Waves I–V. The differential effect of rate on various components of the ABR suggests the presence of peripheral and central rate effects. More rapid stimulus rates also tend to reduce the clarity and reproducibility of responses, particularly for the earlier components. Figure 2–6 shows ABRs obtained in a normal-hearing subject at rates of 7.7, 27.7, 57.7, and 77.7 per second.

Comparison of ABRs obtained at high rates to those obtained at slower presentation rates is sometimes used to evaluate suspected neurological lesions (Don et al., 1977; Stockard, Stockard, & Sharbrough, 1978; see Case Study 7). Rate effects are less reliable than latency as a comparison parameter and, therefore, more difficult to interpret. Because Wave V shows less of an amplitude decrease at high rates, evaluation at high rates can sometimes also serve to identify Wave V in difficult to evaluate tracings. For the same reason, faster rates can be used in threshold-seeking procedures where only the presence or absence of Wave V is of interest. This issue is further discussed in Chapter 6 in relation to use of the ABR to estimate hearing sensitivity.

4.1.3. Stimulus Polarity

Stimulus polarities for ABR testing can be selected as rarefaction, condensation, or alternating between rarefaction and condensation stimuli. Because latencies of the various components in the resulting response are dependent on the polarity of the test stimuli, both consistent use of a particular polarity when comparing results to normative data or previous tests and knowledge of the effects of polarity are critical.

4.1.3.1. Rarefaction Stimuli

A rarefaction stimulus produces an initial outward movement of the earphone diaphragm that generally leads to an outward movement of the footplate of the stapes and an upward motion of the basalmost structures of the organ of Corti. Because the upward motion of the basilar membrane is the depolarizing motion for the hair cells, latency is slightly shorter and amplitude is higher for the early components of the ABR for rarefaction pulses in comparison to condensation pulses in the majority of individuals (Borg & Lofqvist, 1982; Coats & Martin, 1977; Kevanishvili & Aphonchenko, 1981; Stockard et al., 1979).

4.1.3.2. Condensation Stimuli

Condensation stimuli produce an initial inward movement, followed by outward movement and depolarization of the hair cells. Thus the early components of the ABR obtained using condensation polarity stimuli may be slightly longer in latency than those produced using rarefaction pulses. Wave V amplitude tends to be larger in response to condensation stimuli for normal-hearing individuals. There is not a significant latency difference in Wave V latency to rarefaction or condensation stimuli in normal individuals (Kevanishvili & Aphonchenko, 1981; Stockard et al., 1979).

4.1.3.3. Alternating Polarity Stimuli

At high intensities, alternating polarity is sometimes used to reduce stimulus artifact. However, alternating-polarity stimuli are *not* recommended for air-conduction testing because spuriously abnormal recordings may result from cancellation of responses that are out of phase, as discussed below. The introduction of insert earphones with an inherent delay line of 0.9 ms has served to reduce the interference of stimulus artifact with the response. Therefore, the only time that alternating-polarity stimuli are recommended is when using a bone-conduction transducer.

4.1.3.4. Polarity and Peripheral Hearing Loss

The effects of polarity on ABRs are particularly important in patients with high-frequency sloping hearing losses. Both studies of patients with high-frequency hearing loss and the use of high-pass masking to simulate hearing loss in normal-hearing persons show considerable latency changes within individuals as a function of polarity. These phase reversals can degrade an ABR sufficiently to interfere with accurate interpretation. Thus in patients with hearing loss, especially high-frequency hearing loss, use of a single polarity stimulus is recommended. In patients with progressively greater high-frequency hearing loss, phase differences are evident for the ABR for condensation versus rarefaction pulses (Coats & Martin, 1977). Simulation of high-frequency hearing loss through high-pass masking indicates that the polarity effects are due primarily to lower frequency contributions to the response that would be particularly apparent in persons with high-frequency hearing loss (Schoonhoven, 1992). Large latency differences between polarities are observed in individual subjects, although there do not seem to be systematic trends when comparisons are made on a group basis (Schoonhoven, 1992; Sininger & Masuda, 1990).

In extreme cases, specific ABR components may be absent for one polarity and present when the other polarity is used (Maurer, 1985). Spurious abnormalities have also been reported in vascular brainstem disease where condensation and rarefaction stimuli yielded quite different brainstem responses (Maurer, Schafer, & Leitner, 1980).

4.1.3.5. Comparison of Rarefaction and Condensation Responses

When a cochlear response or stimulus artifact is large, as in the case of supra-aural earphones, it can be reduced by separately acquiring responses using rarefaction stimuli and responses using condensation stimuli. If comparison of these responses shows that the ABR waveform components are either in phase or only slightly out of phase, then they can be digitally added together to reduce the cochlear response or the stimulus artifact, improve the signal-to-noise ratio, and elucidate the early components of the ABR. This method is illustrated in Figure 4–1.

There is also a group of patients in whom ABRs may appear to be present when in fact the acquired waves represent the cochlear potential (Berlin, 1996; Berlin et al., 1998). In these patients, the latency does *not* increase as the intensity of the stimulus is decreased, which is the first indication that this is not a neural response. When the polarity of the click is reversed, the waves also invert, con-

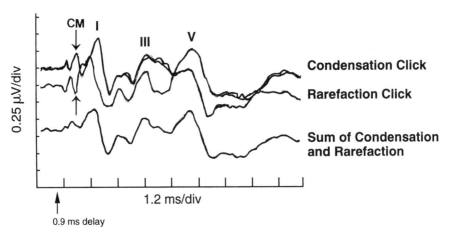

Figure 4–1. Condensation and rarefaction traces and digital sum of the two in a case with an ABR present. The cochlear response (prior to Wave I) reverses in polarity and is nearly completely reduced when the condensation and rarefaction waveforms are summed. The ABR peaks show slight latency differences but remain present in the summed tracing. CM = cochlear microphonic.

sistent with the cochlear microphonic, as shown in Figure 4–2. This finding has been observed in a number of infants with normal otoacoustic emissions and an apparent auditory neuropathy (Berlin et al., 1998; see Case Study 17). Comparing separate averages of both rarefaction and condensation stimuli will aid in identification of patients with auditory neuropathy, and, as discussed later, this procedure is now a part of our standard ABR protocol.

4.1.4. Stimulus Duration and Rise Time

The standard pulse duration utilized in clinical ABR testing is 100 microseconds or 0.1 ms. Because the ABR is an onset response, the duration of the stimulus should not alter the response (Hecox, Squires, & Galambos, 1976; Stapells & Picton, 1981).

There are some special applications where a stimulus with a different duration may be desirable. Examples include testing higher frequency regions of the cochlea to monitor ototoxicity effects and testing patients who exhibit severe hearing losses across the standard audiometric frequency range and normal or nearly normal high-frequency hearing between 8000 and 16,000 Hz (Berlin, Wexler, Jerger, Halperin, & Smith, 1978). A 100-microsecond pulse creates a null in the spectrum at 1/pulse width or 10,000 Hz, whereas a 50-microsecond pulse will not create a null until 20,000 Hz. Therefore, a 50-microsecond pulse is recommended with a suitable transducer (such as Etymotic Research ER-2 or Koss HV/

X earphones) to assess responses in frequency regions of the cochlea responsive to stimuli above 8000 Hz.

In contrast to duration, the rise time of the stimulus has a marked effect on the ABR that is related to reduced synchrony due to fewer neurons firing simultaneously. As rise time increases, latency increases, amplitude decreases, and the morphology deteriorates. Rise times greater than 5 ms may fail to generate a brainstem response. This topic is further discussed in Chapter 6 in Section 6.4.

4.1.5. Stimulus Frequency

The ABR can be obtained using tonebursts that have a rapid rise time while still maintaining some frequency specificity (Picton, Oullette, Hamel, & Smith, 1979). There is a trade-off between frequency specificity and neural synchrony in that tonebursts with longer rise times will be more frequency specific, but will generate poorer neural synchrony, which will affect the quality of the response. Recommended toneburst stimuli are discussed in greater detail in Chapter 6 in relation to the evaluation of hearing sensitivity using the ABR.

Higher frequency stimuli elicit shorter latencies than lower frequency stimuli because high frequencies stimulate the more basal portions of the basilar membrane. This generates earlier responses because the traveling wave moves from the base to the apex. Lower frequency stimuli are analyzed later and in a

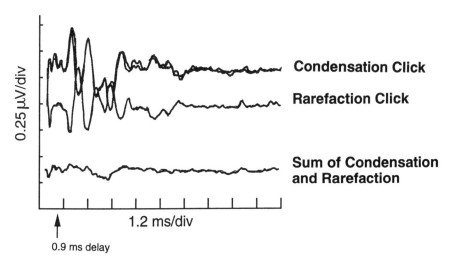

Figure 4-2. Condensation and rarefaction traces and digital sum of the two in a case with no ABR. The cochlear response reverses in polarity and is nearly completely reduced when the condensation and rarefaction waveforms are summed. No ABR is observed in the summed tracing.

less synchronous manner than high-frequency stimuli, resulting in less distinct waveforms.

4.1.6. Monaural Versus Binaural Recordings

Responses to binaural stimuli show an average of a 60% increase in amplitude over responses recorded using monaural stimuli (Blegvad, 1975). Latencies of responses obtained with monaural or binaural stimuli should be similar. Although binaural stimuli may be used as part of the test battery (e.g., in initial averages to evaluate hearing sensitivity as discussed in Chapter 6), monaural stimuli should always be included to assess the function of each ear individually. When using binaural stimuli for either neurological or hearing evaluation in the presence of a unilateral disorder, the response usually reflects only the response of the more normal ear and thus will not reveal the presence of a unilateral disorder.

Comparison of and digital subtraction of recordings obtained from monaural versus binaural stimulation led to the description of the binaural interaction component (BIC) of the ABR, which reflects amplitude and phase differences between monaural and binaural stimulus conditions (Dobie & Berlin, 1979). The fact that the binaural response is not the same as the sum of the monaural responses indicates differences in the response of the auditory system to binaural versus monaural stimuli. A number of studies have addressed the characteristics and generators of binaural interaction components of auditory evoked potentials (e.g., Dobie & Norton, 1980; Gardi & Berlin, 1981; McPherson & Starr, 1993; Polyakov & Pratt, 1995) and the BIC is used as a research tool. The binaural interaction component has not as yet achieved widespread clinical application.

4.2. EFFECTS OF RECORDING FACTORS

4.2.1. Electrode Montages

Placement of electrodes at the vertex (C_z) and ears (A_1 and A_2) and recording between the vertex and ear (C_z–A_1 for the left side and C_z–A_2 for the right side) is optimum for recording the ABR in most conditions (Martin & Moore, 1977; Terkildsen et al., 1975). Waves I–III are more prominent in ipsilateral recordings, whereas Waves IV and V often are better separated in contralateral recordings (Mizrahi, Maulsby, & Frost, 1983).

Earlobe sites tend to result in less muscle potential and greater Wave I amplitude than mastoid recording sites (Stockard & Stockard, 1981). Use of a noncephalic site (such as C_7—the seventh cervical vertebra) may enhance the amplitude of Waves V, VI, and SN_{10}. Ear-to-ear (horizontal) recordings show a reduction in Wave V amplitude while preserving Wave I amplitude.

4.2.2. Filter Settings

When speaking of filtering and filter characteristics related to the recording of the ABR, one is describing the filter band through which the *physiological response* is recorded from the electrodes. This is distinguished from any filtering of a stimulus transduced through an earphone. Filtering of the physiological response is used to eliminate as much internal noise (e.g., unrelated muscle potentials) and external electrical noise (e.g., 60 Hz) as possible. The filters are set to pass the signal of interest, in this case the ABR.

Changes in the frequency band through which the physiological response is filtered affect waveform latency and amplitude. Increasing the high-pass filter cutoff frequency (i.e., reducing the low-frequency energy) from 30 Hz to 100 or 150 Hz results in decreases in the amplitude and latency of the response. Allowing more low-frequency information into the average generally results in increased amplitude, particularly for the later components, and slightly longer latencies. Decreasing the low-pass filter cutoff frequency (e.g., from 3000 Hz to 1500 Hz) may result in some rounding of the peaks, but has less effect on amplitude or latency. Examples of ABRs acquired with various filter bands are shown in Figure 4–3.

Interference from electrical sources and muscle activity increases as more low frequencies are included. Wave V amplitude may increase because it is dependent on the amount of low-frequency energy included due to direct current (DC) offset and the low-frequency components of Wave V. Use of very narrow filters is discouraged because phase shifting may occur in frequency regions near the cutoff frequencies.

4.2.3. Time Window

The time window, or analysis time, should be set to encompass all components of the response. The length of the time window will vary with the age of the patient and the intensity and type of stimulus used. For presentation of click stimuli in adult patients, a time window of 10 or 12 ms is usually sufficient to record the ABR because Wave V occurs in normal individuals within 5 to 6 ms of the stimulus at high intensities and within 8 to 9 ms for intensities near threshold. Use of insert earphones will delay the response by slightly less than 1 ms, which is still within a 10-ms time frame. In infants ABR components are delayed by 1 ms or more; therefore a time window of at least 15 ms is recommended when testing patients below 18 months of age or in patients older than 18 months if delays in neuromaturation are suspected.

Although a 10- to 15-ms time window is sufficient when using click stimuli, ABR testing with tonebursts requires a time window of at least 20 ms. This is particu-

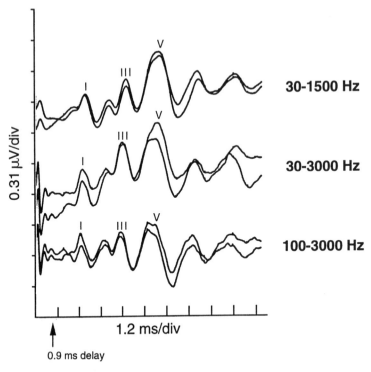

Figure 4–3. ABRs obtained with three different filter settings. Responses are present for all three filter settings, but may show differences in amplitude, generally with increased amplitude as more low-frequency energy is included.

larly true when using 250- or 500-Hz tonebursts where the stimuli have a longer onset time and activate more apical portions of the cochlear partition. Issues related to the use of toneburst stimuli are discussed in Chapter 6.

One instance where it may be necessary to shorten the time window is in patients who have a large postauricular muscle (PAM) artifact, which may occur in the 8- to 12-ms time range. The PAM artifact usually occurs with higher intensity stimuli and may cause the artifact rejection system to reject all sweeps. In this case, it may help to shorten the time window to about 8 ms, as long as Wave V is still visible. As an alternative, the clinician may disable the artifact rejection system in quiet patients and monitor the input signal manually. An example of an ABR with a PAM artifact is shown in Figure 4–4 and in Case Study 19.

4.2.4. One- Versus Two-Channel Recordings

Two-channel recording instruments allow acquisition of both ipsilateral and contralateral recordings simultaneously. Generally, this is the preferred method for obtaining ABRs. In single-channel instruments, it is possible to collect ipsilateral

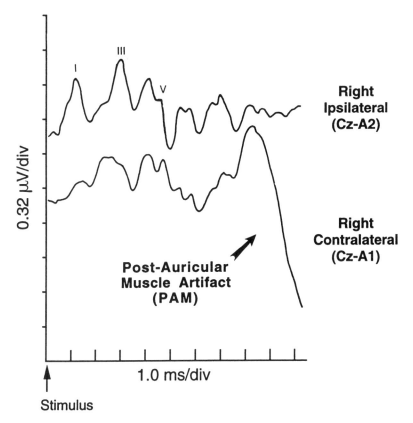

Figure 4-4. Example of a patient with a postauricular muscle artifact (noted by the arrow) in the right contralateral waveform.

and contralateral ABRs in sequential runs, one while recording from the electrode montage ipsilateral to the ear being stimulated (e.g., $C_z–A_1$ for stimulation of the left ear), followed by changing the electrode hookup and recording from the contralateral electrode montage while stimulating the same ear as before (e.g., $C_z–A_2$ for stimulation of the left ear).

There are several reasons to obtain simultaneous two-channel recordings whenever possible. Obtaining both responses allows the examiner to accomplish the following:

1. Avoid electrode misrouting errors that occur in one-channel recordings when the operator either forgets to change the ear electrode or incorrectly assigns it.
2. Monitor the ear that was stimulated by the amplitude of the artifact in the response and position of the trace containing Wave I.
3. Determine the presence and location of Wave I by comparison to the contralateral recording. Wave I should not be present in the contralateral tracing.

4. Obtain better definition of Waves IV and V because they tend to be more separated in contralateral recordings.
5. Subtract contralateral from ipsilateral recordings to derive a horizontal recording, which may assist in distinguishing Wave I.
6. Examine the integrity of each cochlea during bone-conduction stimulation because finding similar Wave I amplitudes for both channels suggests that stimuli are being transduced through both cochleae.

4.2.5. Number of Sweeps

The number of sweeps required in an averaged response varies according to the inherent amplitude of the evoked potential and the amount of background noise, which can include muscle artifact, 60-Hz noise, electroencephalographic (EEG) activity, and so forth. For the ABR, usually 1000 to 2000 sweeps are adequate to obtain clear responses in quiet patients when using higher intensity stimuli. At lower intensities where the response amplitude is lower, more sweeps may be necessary to achieve an adequate signal-to-noise ratio.

As shown in Chapter 3 in Figure 3–2, the amount of improvement in the signal-to-noise ratio varies with the number of sweeps. Once a certain number of sweeps are included in an average, addition of further data may provide minimal benefit in improving the signal-to-noise ratio. Use of objective estimates of the signal-to-noise ratio, such as F_{SP}, is very helpful in determining the number of sweeps required to obtain the best possible response.

4.3. EFFECTS OF PATIENT FACTORS

4.3.1. Age

The ABR changes as a function of age, particularly during the first 12 to 18 months of life, as the central auditory system continues to mature. Characteristics of ABRs obtained in premature and term infants vary from those obtained in adults (Hecox & Galambos, 1974; Jacobson, Morehouse, & Johnson, 1982; Schulman-Galambos & Galambos, 1975; Starr, Amlie, Martin, & Sanders, 1977). Reliable ABR components for 65-dB nHL clicks have been reported in newborns of approximately 28 weeks gestational age (Starr et al., 1977). Waves I, III, and V are most visible in infant recordings and the normal Wave V absolute latency for a newborn approximates 7.0 ms at 60 dB nHL. The amplitude of Waves I and/or III may be greater than Wave V in infants. Responses obtained from infants 12 to

18 months of age and older should resemble those acquired from adults (Hecox & Galambos, 1974; Salamy, McKean, & Buda, 1975).

Wave I may be slightly prolonged in infants, but generally is not as prolonged as Wave V. This results in a longer interwave latency of about 5.0 ms compared to 4.0 ms in adults (Hecox & Galambos, 1974; Starr et al., 1977). This prolongation may be related to cochlear maturation (Rubel & Ryals, 1983; Ryan, Woolf, & Sharp, 1982), neuronal maturation (Starr et al., 1977; Stockard & Stockard, 1981), reduced efficiency in external and/or middle ear sound transmission, and occasionally collapsing ear canals. Recent reports suggest that neural maturation of the auditory system is complex, with conduction time adultlike by term birth, pathway lengthening continuing to mature until about age 3 years, and different aspects of myelin development contributing to changes in ABRs in infants (Moore, Ponton, Eggermont, Wu, & Huang, 1996).

Absence of an ABR to 85-dB nHL stimuli is reported in some infants who later develop normally or in infants with neurological disease (Kraus, Özdamar, Stein, & Reed, 1984; Stockard & Stockard, 1981; Worthington & Peters, 1980). Use of otoacoustic emissions as part of the test battery can distinguish infants with normal peripheral function from those with neurological disease. Presentation of test stimuli at rates over 60 per second or use of maximum length sequence (MLS) methods also may desynchronize the waveform, giving the appearance of an absent response (Stockard & Stockard, 1981) or greater Wave V prolongation than expected (Fujikawa & Weber, 1977; Salamy et al., 1975).

The effects of age on the ABR in adults is less clear. Adults 55 years of age and older have demonstrated 0.1 to 0.2 ms longer latencies than adults aged 20 to 30 years in some studies (Allison, Wood, & Goff, 1983; Jerger & Hall, 1980; Otto & McCandless, 1982; Rowe, 1978). Other studies have shown no significant age effects in subjects from 10 to 60 years of age (Beagley & Sheldrake, 1978; Stockard & Stockard, 1981; Stockard et al., 1979). In addition, there appears to be an interaction of age and gender. For example, greater increases in Wave V latency with age have been reported in males than in females (Jerger & Johnson, 1988).

4.3.2. Gender

Females tend to have shorter latency and higher amplitude ABRs than males (Allison et al., 1983; Beagley & Sheldrake, 1978; Elberling & Parbo, 1987; Jerger & Hall, 1980; Kjaer, 1979; Michalewski, Thompson, Patterson, Bowman, & Litzelman, 1980; Stockard, Stockard, & Sharbrough, 1978; Watson, 1996). Wave V latency averages about 0.2 ms shorter in females, and amplitude is higher in females, particularly for Waves IV, V, VI, and VII. Females may also show shorter interwave latencies than males. It has been suggested that the source of the differences in latency and amplitude in the ABR between males and females may be related to shorter cochlear response times in females than males (Don, Ponton, Eggermont, & Masuda, 1994).

4.3.3. Age and Gender

When age and gender in adults are considered together, the shortest latencies are obtained from younger females, with latency increasing for older females, then younger males, and finally, the longest latencies are recorded from older males (Stockard, Stockard, & Sharbrough, 1978). Elberling and Parbo (1987) compared the effects of age, gender, and hearing loss on the Waves I–V interwave latency and reported that, for subjects with normal hearing, the mean interwave latency increased from 4.0 ms for 20- to 30-year-old females to 4.2 ms for female subjects from 70–80 years. A slightly greater increase with age was observed in male subjects, where the interwave latency of Waves I–V increased from 4.2 ms for 20- to 30-year-old males to 4.5 ms for 70- to 80-year-old males.

4.3.4. Medication

Studies suggest that the ABR is not influenced by sedatives, relaxants, barbiturates, or anesthesia (Sanders, Duncan, & McCullough, 1979; Starr, 1977). However, abnormal ABRs have been reported in conjunction with medications such as phenytoin, lidocaine, and diazepam. Also, carbamazepine (CBZ) monotherapy in epileptic patients has been reported to result in prolongation of the peak latencies of Waves I, III, and V and prolongation of Waves I–III and I–V intervals (Japaridze, Kvernadze, Geladze, & Kevanishvili, 1993). Documentation of medications should assist in appropriate interpretation of test results.

The ABR can be useful in monitoring the effects of ototoxic drugs. Click stimuli transduced through standard earphones, which provide maximum stimulation in the 2000 to 4000 Hz range, may pick up losses when they appear in that frequency range. High-frequency tonebursts at 8000 Hz and above transduced through special earphones may be even more sensitive to the effects of aminoglycosides because higher frequency sensitivity is often affected first. The ABR also offers particular utility because it does not require behavioral responses from patients and thus can be performed on ill patients (Guerit, Mahieu, Houben-Giurgea, & Herbay, 1981).

4.3.5. Attention

ABR recordings do not appear to be affected by sleep (Jewett & Williston, 1971), are not altered by metabolic or toxic coma (Starr, 1977), and do not differ significantly for clinical purposes as a function of attention (Picton & Hillyard, 1974). The lack of effects from sleep and medication enhance the utility of the ABR in a wide variety of patient populations.

4.3.6. Body Temperature

As body temperature increases or decreases from the normal range, shifts in absolute peak latencies have been observed. Jones, Stockard, and Weidner (1980) reported a correlation between rises in body temperature and decreases in latency in cats. Stockard, Sharbrough, and Tinker (1978) reported a correlation between decreases in esophageal temperature (below 35° C) and increases in interpeak latency of Waves I–V. Because of these temperature effects, care should be taken to document temperature during intraoperative monitoring procedures and when evaluating comatose patients (Stockard, Rossiter, Jones, & Sharbrough, 1977).

Latency increases have also been observed with alcohol intake, which is most likely related to decreases in body temperature. Prolonged acute alcohol intoxication or chronic alcohol use can result in prolongation of Wave V (Chu, Squires, & Starr, 1978; Squires, Chu, & Starr, 1978).

4.3.7. Muscle Artifact

The ABR is minimally affected by myogenic potentials (muscle activity), although a quiet patient state generally facilitates detection of responses, particularly at intensity levels near threshold. Excessive muscle artifact often arises from the jaw or neck muscles. Thus, ensuring that patients are resting comfortably with their heads well supported and their jaws unclenched can facilitate acquisition of quality recordings.

Occasionally patients may display spontaneous nystagmus when they close their eyes. Because eye movement may result in muscle artifact that interferes with ABR recording, patients with nystagmus should be advised to open their eyes and fixate on an object.

PART II

Clinical Applications of the Auditory Brainstem Response

Clinical Applications of the ABR in Neurological Testing

This chapter describes auditory brainstem response (ABR) test protocols used in neurological evaluations and the characteristics of ABRs in individuals with various neural disorders. Although protocols vary among centers, the following discussion is intended to represent both a composite overview of methods and some of our own practices for each type of evaluation.

5.1. APPLICATION AND PROCEDURE

The ABR is used in neurological testing for differential diagnosis. It can be used to assist in determination of the presence or absence of a disorder and, to a limited extent, the site of a disorder. In the auditory system, it is necessary to distinguish a cochlear from a more central lesion, such as along the eighth nerve or brainstem pathways. The ABR is also useful in combination with other tests in the identification of diffuse lesions, such as those associated with multiple sclerosis, and disorders that are not associated with a radiologically identifiable lesion, such as auditory neuropathy.

5.1.1. Who Should Be Tested?

Patients who report dizziness, unilateral tinnitus, asymmetric hearing loss, sudden-onset hearing loss, or progressive hearing loss are good candidates for ABR evaluation, as are those who report dizziness or tinnitus with no hearing difficulty. Patients with unexplained elevation or absence of middle ear muscle reflexes (MEMRs), unexplained unilateral hearing loss, abnormally poor word recognition in quiet, reduced word recognition in noise, and/or PIPB rollover are also good candidates for ABR evaluation.

5.1.2. Test Procedures

Click stimuli are presented at a level well above threshold (usually between 70 and 90 dB nHL) to each ear individually. Initial rates of stimulus presentation ranging from approximately 10 to 30 stimuli per second are used to obtain baseline information. Presentation rates such as 11.1 or 27.7 stimuli per second are used to avoid repetition rates that are multiples of 60 Hz that could introduce power-line artifact into the response. When clear responses are not obtained at these rates, the presentation rate should be decreased below 10 per second (e.g., 7.7 per second). If clear responses are not obtained at the initial test intensity, then the intensity of the stimuli may be increased to further define responses. Care should be taken not to exceed the patient's maximum comfort levels for the test stimuli. Using the standard click ABR test parameters shown in Table 5–1, a recommended test protocol is shown in Table 5–2.

Table 5-1. Test parameters for air-conduction click ABR for neurological evaluation.

Test Parameter	Setting
Stimulus	100 μs click
Stimulus polarity	Condensation Rarefaction
Stimulus rate	27.7/s
Stimulus intensity	75 dB nHL or higher as needed
Time window	10 or 12 ms
Filter bandwidth	100–3000 Hz
Number of channels	Two
Electrode montage	C_Z–A_1 and C_Z–A_2
Number of sweeps	1500–2000
Number of replications	Two

Table 5-2. Test protocol for neurological application of the ABR.

Parameter	Setting/Action
Stimulus	Air-conduction clicks
Stimulus intensity	75 dB nHL (or higher as necessary)
Stimulus rate	Begin at 27.7/s
Fast stimulus rate	57.7/s or 77.7/s
To enhance Wave I	Decrease stimulus rate Increase stimulus intensity Use ear canal or tympanic electrode Electrocochleography
If no Wave I obtained	Toneburst at highest frequency where hearing thresholds are symmetric (e.g., 1000 Hz or 1500 Hz)

Generally, between 1000 and 2000 sweeps are averaged together to provide a sufficient number of responses for interpretation, and each test condition is repeated to ensure replicability of responses. Presentation of stimuli at a rate higher than 50 per second and a latency-intensity series also may be included in neurological evaluation.

5.1.3. Identification of Wave I

A common diagnostic problem, particularly when testing persons with high-frequency hearing loss, is difficulty in identifying Wave I. Wave I identification is usually necessary to determine interwave latency intervals for Waves I–III and I–V. Wave V latency to a 75-dB nHL signal of 6.0 ms or less that is symmetric with the response from the other ear generally represents a normal ABR, although exceptions do occur. In this case, a specific Wave I latency is less necessary to ensure a normal Waves I–V interval. Because Wave I at 75 dB nHL does not routinely occur at less than 1.4 to 1.6 ms, a 4.4- to 4.6-ms Waves I–V interval is the worst case that could result when Wave V latency is 6.0 ms or less. However, for correct interpretation, these ABRs should be closely examined for any abnormalities or asymmetries and efforts still should be made to obtain a Wave I.

Methods used to increase apparent Wave I amplitude include (a) increasing the intensity of the stimulus, (b) decreasing the presentation rate, (c) comparing rarefaction and condensation clicks to distinguish cochlear potentials from neural responses, (d) using electrocochleography (ECochG) where an electrode is placed near the cochlea (e.g., on the promontory in the middle ear or in the ear canal near the eardrum), and (e) using a horizontal recording montage where recordings are obtained between the electrodes at the respective ear lobes (A_1 and A_2).

Use of ear canal electrodes, particularly those placed at or near the tympanic membrane, combines ECochG procedures to delineate the early components with ABR recording in order to quantify the Waves I–V interval. This can provide a useful clinical procedure in cases where identification of Wave I is difficult (e.g., Ferraro & Ferguson, 1989). Brantberg (1996) reported on 50 patients with unilateral auditory signs who had a delayed Wave V in the symptomatic ear and an absence of Wave I in that ear. With the use of an ear canal electrode an identifiable Wave I was obtained in 72% of the cases.

5.1.4. Use of Masking

When there are significant sensitivity differences between the two ears, masking is recommended for the opposite ear (Clemis & Mitchell, 1977; Humes & Ochs, 1982; Özdamar & Stein, 1981; see Case Study 8). Ideally one could avoid masking in most cases by using insert phones (Killion, 1984). If masking is needed, then a broadband noise is the best masker when using a click stimulus because the click spectrum encompasses a broad frequency range. The rules that apply to the need for masking and the amount of masking to be used are similar to the rules that apply to conventional audiometric pure-tone testing where both air-conduction and bone-conduction thresholds must be known.

5.2. EFFECTS OF COCHLEAR HEARING LOSS

The degree of peripheral hearing loss and the configuration of the loss can affect the ability to obtain an ABR, the definition of the waveform components, and the latency and amplitude parameters. However, the degree of hearing loss should *never* preclude an attempt to obtain an ABR (see Case Study 8).

5.2.1. Wave V Latency

Normal Wave V latencies have been observed at stimulus levels of 70 to 90 dB nHL in patients with Ménière's disease and hearing losses of up to 60 dB HL (Galambos & Hecox, 1978; Picton et al., 1977; see Case 1). Bauch and Olsen (1986, 1987) reported that Wave V latency and waveform morphology were progressively affected by greater degrees of peripheral hearing loss as well as by increasing slopes of hearing loss. In their series of 458 patients, they obtained normal ABRs in nearly all of the patients whose hearing sensitivity was normal through 2000 Hz and better than 35 dB HL at 3000 and 4000 Hz. When hearing loss at 4000 Hz exceeded 50 dB HL, Wave I was often absent, and when thresholds from 2000–4000 Hz were in the 50 to 70 dB HL range, the number of abnormal ABRs increased rapidly. Patients with sharply downward sloping audiograms (i.e., greater high-frequency hearing loss) showed Wave V delays, which may be related to stimulation of fewer basal and more apical regions of the cochlea.

Patients with rising audiograms, especially those with best hearing from 2000 to 4000 Hz, are more likely to yield normal ABRs. When averages of 2000, 3000, and 4000 Hz were obtained, 72% of the ABRs were normal for pure-tone averages of 50–59 dB HL (Bauch & Olsen, 1987). Even with pure-tone averages of 70–79 dB HL, 41% of the ABRs were judged normal.

5.2.2. Latency-Intensity Functions in Cochlear Hearing Losses

Predictable latency changes occur with alterations in intensity, and some components of the response should be observed at levels within 15 to 20 dB of behavioral threshold. With some limitations, the ABR provides information about peripheral hearing and can be used to distinguish among different types of hearing loss. This application of the ABR is discussed in Chapter 6.

The latency-intensity function observed in cochlear hearing loss is often steeper than that seen in persons with normal hearing or conductive or retrocochlear hearing loss (Coats, 1978; see Figure 5–1). This occurs because Wave V latency increases at faster than normal rates at moderate intensities. As the intensity of the stimulus increases, response amplitude also increases more rapidly in subjects with cochlear hearing loss than in normal-hearing subjects. In patients with high-frequency hearing loss, Wave V latency increases, requiring a greater intensity level before a Wave V can be identified (Coats & Martin, 1977; Møller & Blegvad, 1976; Yamada, Kodera, & Yagi, 1979).

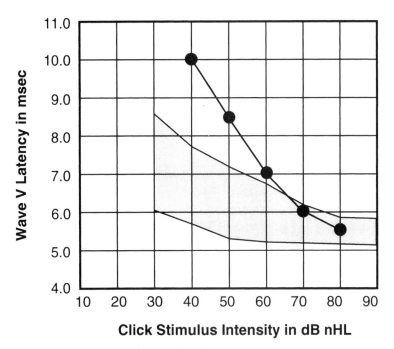

Figure 5-1. Wave V latency-intensity function observed in a patient with a cochlear hearing loss. At lower intensities, absolute Wave V latency is longer than normal, but is within the normal range when clicks are presented at higher intensities.

5.2.3. High-Frequency Hearing Loss

Subjects with steep high-frequency hearing loss sometimes also show a reduced I-V interpeak latency interval (Coats, 1978) because Wave I is prolonged more than Wave V. The Waves I–V interval has been reported to decrease progressively with increased cochlear hearing loss in the higher frequencies (Elberling and Parbo, 1987). Although these changes were constant across age, males showed a greater decrease than females, with increasing hearing loss in the Waves I–V interval.

5.2.4. Asymmetric Hearing Loss

Because most eighth nerve tumors, with the exception of those in patients with neurofibromatosis, are unilateral, asymmetric hearing losses often result. If the hearing loss is less than approximately 60 dB HL and cochlear in origin, then normal ABRs to high-intensity clicks are the usual result (see Case Study 1 in Chapter 8). Stimuli that are approximately 20 dB higher than thresholds in the 2000 to 4000 Hz range are often sufficient for the recruitment effect to overcome the effect of the hearing loss (Durrant & Fowler, 1996). If it is not possible to present stimuli at 20 dB above the threshold of a cochlear hearing loss, then latencies may not attain normal values.

5.2.5. Stimulus Polarity Interactions With Cochlear Hearing Loss

The polarity of the stimulus used in recording the ABR may interact with the obtained response. Use of alternating-polarity stimuli can result in cancellation of the response due to the recording of components that are out of phase (Coats & Martin, 1977; Stockard & Stockard, 1981). Therefore, we recommend the use of either condensation or rarefaction clicks individually and *do not* recommend the use of alternating-polarity stimuli. If the stimulus artifact is large, then it may be desirable to acquire responses to condensation clicks and store them in one computer memory and acquire responses to rarefaction clicks and store them in another memory. Then, following inspection of the responses and determination that there are *not* large latency shifts with polarity changes, the two sets of responses can be added together to reduce the stimulus artifact. Use of insert earphones reduces the contamination of the response by stimulus artifact.

5.2.6. Overcoming the Effects of Peripheral Hearing Loss

Perhaps one of the greatest limitations and frustrations in using the ABR occurs in the evaluation of patients with substantial peripheral hearing loss. The effectiveness of the stimulus is decreased by peripheral hearing loss, impairing clear definition of waveforms, particularly earlier components, which may cloud the interpretation of differences between ears.

5.2.6.1. Identification of Wave I

Identification of Wave I latency will allow calculation of the Waves I-V interval and resolve whether the reason for the Wave I delay is related to peripheral hearing loss or a retrocochlear lesion. Enhancement of Wave I can be accomplished by parametric changes such as decreasing stimulus rate, increasing stimulus intensity, using an ear canal or tympanic electrode, or transtympanic ECochG. Tympanic or transtympanic electrodes will yield the largest Wave I and generally are most useful in distinguishing Wave I in these difficult cases. If any synchronous activity is present in the early latency period, then reversing the polarity of the stimulus is useful in distinguishing the location of the cochlear response (cochlear microphonic) and differentiating it from neural activity (i.e., Wave I).

5.2.6.2. Correction Factors

Some clinicians recommend the use of correction factors for hearing loss, although this should be approached with caution. For example, Selters and Brackmann (1979) recommended subtracting 0.1 ms from the Wave V latency for every 10-dB threshold increase above 50 dB HL at 4000 Hz. In one study, use of this correction factor in patients with hearing loss greater than 50 dB at 4000 Hz showed a decrease in false-positive results with the correction factor, but a slight increase in the false-negative rate (Cashman, Stanton, Sagle, & Barber, 1993).

There are additional methods, which may be more direct in addressing the problem, that can be used to acquire responses to assist in interpretation. The most direct method is to try to enhance Wave I, using the procedures previously described.

5.2.6.3. Alternative Methods

Another method of overcoming the effects of high-frequency hearing loss, particularly asymmetric loss, utilizes midfrequency tonebursts where hearing is more symmetric. In these patients, the highest frequency where hearing is fairly normal and symmetric between ears may yield better synchrony than where hearing loss is substantial and thus allow acquisition of more useful information than possible with a click stimulus. Telian and Kileny (1989) recommended the use of 1000-Hz tonebursts in each ear when hearing is relatively normal or symmetric between the two ears in this frequency range. Although Waves I and III may not be obtained, it should be possible to record a Wave V if the loss is cochlear in nature and to compare the Wave V latencies for each ear. If the latencies are similar, then it is more likely that the loss is cochlear in origin.

For ABRs obtained using 1000-Hz tonebursts, interaural latency differences tend to be more variable among patients with sensory (cochlear) hearing loss for tonebursts than for clicks, and relatively unaffected by hearing asymmetries above 1000 Hz (Gorga, Kaminski, Beauchaine, & Schulte, 1992). Although the improvement in test sensitivity and specificity obtained by adding the 1000-Hz toneburst condition to the test battery may appear limited, it can provide a useful confirmatory measure (Campbell & Brady, 1995).

Generally ABRs are compared between ears for stimuli presented at equal intensity levels. In cases where there are significant differences in sensitivity and toneburst recordings cannot be obtained, another alternative method that may be useful is to compare responses obtained at intensities that are balanced in loudness between the two ears. In this case, the patient is asked to report when stimuli are equally loud in each ear. Practically, the stimuli presented through earphones will lateralize toward the ear where the stimulus is louder when there is an imbalance in loudness. When stimuli are equally loud in each ear, a single stimulus should be heard in the center of the head. In our practice, we have found it useful to have the patient simply point to the place on the head where he or she hears the stimulus. When the clicks are equal in loudness, the patient should point to the center of the head. Following this determination of equally loud intensity levels, ABRs can be obtained at these two intensities and Wave V latencies compared for symmetry of responses from the two ears.

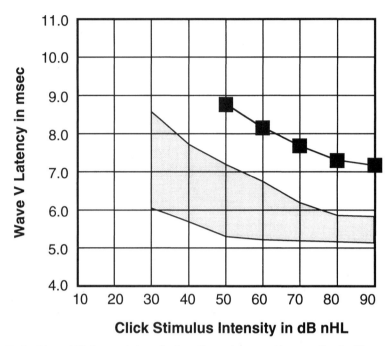

Figure 5-2. Wave V latency-intensity function observed in a patient with a conductive hearing loss. Absolute Wave V latencies are longer than normal for all intensities.

The clinician should approach all of these alternative methods with caution because there may exist unknown interactions with the nature and configuration of the hearing loss. However, when data are difficult to interpret or uninterpretable, the additional information may prove useful in conjunction with the other audiological and medical findings.

5.3. EFFECTS OF CONDUCTIVE HEARING LOSS

Conductive hearing loss results in a prolongation of all waves; with interpeak intervals remaining within normal limits (see Case Studies 12 and 13). The Wave V latency-intensity function is shifted from the normal range for all stimulus intensities (Figure 5–2). The shift in latency of the entire waveform is a result of the reduction in the level of the signal arriving at the cochlea by the conductive hearing loss. The amount that the latency-intensity function for click stimuli is offset from the normal latency-intensity function is generally consistent with the amount of conductive hearing loss in the higher frequencies (Fria & Sabo, 1980).

Wave I prolongation has been reported in otitis media, with a return to normal values after the otitis resolved (Mendelson, Salamy, Lenoir, & McKean, 1979). Wave V latency-intensity functions are reported to correlate well with ear canal occlusion and middle ear effusion, but not ossicular chain disorders (McGee & Clemis, 1982).

Recent reports also suggest that long-term effects of otitis media with effusion (OME) may affect the ABR even after hearing sensitivity has returned to normal. Hall and Grose (1993) compared children with and without a history of otitis media and found that children with a history of OME had significantly prolonged Waves III and V and prolonged I–III and I–V intervals. These results, along with abnormal masking level differences, suggest the possibility of some type of abnormal brainstem processing in the group with a history of OME.

Failure to place supra-aural earphones over the ear canals, shifts in the earphones resulting from patient movement, and collapse of the ear canals as a result of pressure from the earphones can all mimic conductive losses and yield spuriously abnormal ABRs. Because Wave V prolongation may also be consistent with a retrocochlear lesion, care must be taken to ensure that earphones are correctly placed and that the ear canals are not collapsed by one or both earphones (see Case Study 18). The widespread use of insert earphones has helped to overcome this problem, and use of insert earphones in evoked potential testing is recommended.

5.4. EFFECTS OF NEUROLOGICAL DISORDERS

The ABR is sensitive to neurological disorders of the eighth nerve and low- to mid-brainstem. These disorders include space-occupying lesions, diffuse lesions, and functional (physiological) abnormalities.

5.4.1. Eighth Nerve Tumors and Other Neoplasms

Tumors along the eighth nerve pathway, such as vestibular schwannomas (also sometimes referred to as acoustic neuromas, neurinomas, or neurilemmomas) and other neoplasms (including meningiomas and gliomas) can result in prolongation of absolute latency, prolongation of interwave latency intervals, degradation of the waveform, and/or absence of waves, particularly the later waves (e.g., Jerger, Mauldin, & Anthony, 1978; Rosenhamer, 1977; Sohmer, Feinmesser, & Szabo, 1974; Starr & Achor, 1975; Starr & Hamilton, 1976; Terkildsen, Huis in't Veld, & Osterhammel, 1977; Thomsen, Terkildsen, & Osterhammel, 1978; Thornton, 1980; see Case Studies 4 through 10). Wave V absolute latency is prolonged at all intensities, as shown in the latency-intensity function in Figure 5–3.

In a series of 61 patients with confirmed eighth nerve or cerebellopontine angle tumors, 30% had no discernible waves, 44% had some waves present (primarily Waves I and/or V), and 26% demonstrated all waves present though latencies were not normal (Musiek, Josey, & Glasscock, 1986). More patients with larger tumors lacked responses, although this observation of a very poor or absent ABR should

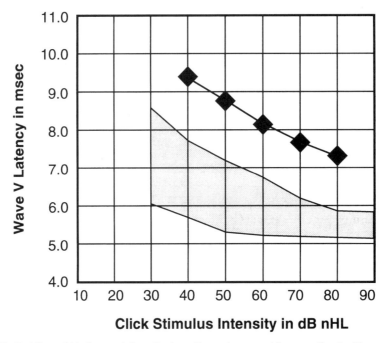

Figure 5-3. Wave V latency-intensity function observed in a patient with a retrocochlear hearing loss. Absolute Wave V latencies are longer than normal for all intensities and the latency-intensity function cannot be distinguished from that obtained with a conductive hearing loss.

not be used to predict tumor size. Also, in cases of large tumors, abnormal recordings from the contralateral side have been reported (Nodar & Kinney, 1980; Shanon, Gold, & Himmelfarb, 1981).

Eighth nerve tumors and auditory brainstem disorders have been observed in patients when the Wave V/I amplitude ratio is less than 0.5 (Starr & Hamilton, 1976), when the latency difference of Wave V between ears is increased beyond 0.4 ms (Selters & Brackmann, 1977; Thomason et al., 1993), and as a result of rate increases (Pratt & Sohmer, 1976). Tumors within the brainstem can also result in degraded waveforms, increased latencies, and absent waves that are generated rostral to the site of the lesion (Jerger et al., 1978; Nodar, Hahn, & Levine, 1980; Starr & Achor, 1975; Starr & Hamilton, 1976; Stockard & Rossiter, 1977). Increasing stimulus rate can result in prolongations in the Waves I-V interval in patients with acoustic tumors beyond that observed in normal individuals (Tanaka, Komatsuzaki, & Hentona, 1996).

Positive identification of tumors by ABR testing has been reported at a rate of 92 to 98% (e.g., Barrs, Brackmann, Olson, & House, 1985; Bauch, Rose, & Harner, 1982; Clemis & McGee, 1979; Eggermont, Don, & Brackmann, 1980; Glasscock, Jackson, Josey, Dickins, & Wiet, 1979; House & Brackmann, 1979). Normal ABRs are most often associated with small tumors (e.g., Bauch, Olsen, & Pool, 1996; Djupesland, Flottorp, Modalsli, Tvete, & Sortland, 1981; G. P. Jacobson, Newman, Monsell, & Wharton, 1993; M. B. Møller & Møller, 1983).

In a retrospective series of 197 patients, a significant difference in sensitivity with respect to tumor size was reported by Chandrasekhar, Brackmann, and Devgan (1996). With ABR interaural latency difference as the measurement parameter, test sensitivity in their series varied from 100% in tumors of 3.0 cm or larger to 83.1% for tumors of 1.0 cm or smaller. In a series of 75 patients, Bauch et al. (1996) found that abnormalities in the Waves I–V interval increased from 77% in patients with tumors smaller than 1.0 cm to 96% in patients with tumors larger than 2.0 cm.

In a prospective study of 105 patients, 87.6% had abnormal ABRs and 12.4% had normal ABRs (Gordon & Cohen, 1995). All 18 patients with tumors larger than 2.5 cm had abnormal ABRs; of 29 patients with tumors 1.6 cm to 2.0 cm, 86% had abnormal ABRs; of 49 patients with tumors 1.0 to 1.5 cm in diameter 89%, had abnormal ABRs; and of 13 patients with tumors 9 mm or smaller, 69% had abnormal ABRs.

Magnetic resonance imaging (MRI) with gadolinium-diethylenetriamine penta-acetic acid (Gd-DTPA) provides a very sensitive diagnostic tool in the identification of eighth nerve tumors (Sidman, Carrasco, Whaley, & Pillsbury, 1989). MRI with Gd-DTPA does not involve radiation or have the side effects that accompany air-contrast computed tomography (CT) and provides sufficient signal enhancement to allow identification of tumors as small as 0.3 cm × 0.3 cm (Stack, Antoun, Jenkins, Metcalfe, & Isherwood, 1988). Some patients in whom tumors are identified by Gd-MRI are asymptomatic, and it is unknown whether these patients would become symptomatic in the future. A number of factors, such as cost and availability, may enter into the determination of whether evaluation of patients suspected to have a tumor in the region of the cerebellopontine angle should begin with ABR or MRI.

5.4.1.1. Normal Pure-Tone Thresholds and Abnormal ABRs

There also have been a number of reports of patients with essentially normal pure-tone thresholds who have abnormal ABRs and acoustic tumors (De Donato, Russo, Taibah, Saleh, & Sanna, 1995; Musiek, Kibbe-Michal, Geurkink, & Josey, 1986; Telian & Kileny, 1988; Valente, Peterein, Goebel, & Neely, 1995; see Case Study 4) or auditory neuropathy (Berlin, Hood, Cecola, Jackson, & Szabo, 1993; Starr, Picton, Sininger, Hood, & Berlin, 1996). By using a combination of absolute and interwave latencies, interaural latency differences, and waveform presence, Musiek, Josey, and Glasscock (1986) found abnormal ABRs in 15 of 16 patients with tumors who had hearing thresholds of 25 dB HL or better between 500 and 4000 Hz. Tumors ranged in size from 0.5 to 4.5 cm, and lesion size failed to correlate with ABR results.

5.4.1.2. Poor Pure-Tone Thresholds and Abnormal ABRs

It also is possible to have very poor pure-tone thresholds with fairly normal cochlear function. This is observed in cases where the hearing loss is related to an effect of the eighth nerve tumor, which may or may not be related to interference with the blood supply to the cochlea (Eggermont et al., 1980). Patients with an auditory neuropathy also may show poor pure-tone thresholds with normal otoacoustic emissions and an absent or markedly abnormal ABR. In cases of auditory neuropathy, otoacoustic emissions and the ABR are a powerful diagnostic combination. In cases of eighth nerve tumors, otoacoustic emissions may or may not be present.

In some cases of severe high-frequency cochlear hearing loss, it may be impossible to obtain an ABR. However, the presence of a severe or even total audiometric loss should not rule out the use of ABR because normal Waves I and II are seen occasionally with patients who have no audiometric response (see Case Study 8). This anomaly is pathognomonic for an eighth nerve lesion near the junction of the eighth nerve into the cochlear nucleus.

5.4.1.3. Neurofibromatosis

Neurofibromatoses fall into two subclasses, neurofibromatosis type 1 (NF1) and neurofibromatosis type 2 (NF2). These are two genetically distinct entities involving the auditory system. NF1 is a multisystem disorder that frequently involves the auditory system. NF2 is characterized by bilateral vestibular schwannomas and is sometimes associated with multiple intracranial and spinal tumors. Auditory system involvement is characterized by abnormal MEMRs and ABRs and testing is useful in both NF1 and NF2 patients and in pediatric as well as adult populations (Pikus, 1995). Most eighth nerve tumors in children have been associated with neurofibromatosis, although cases have been reported of children with a vestibular schwannoma not associated with neurofibromatosis (e.g., Sells & Hurley, 1994).

5.4.1.4. Strategies in Interpretation of Results in Patients with Suspected Tumors

There are a number of ABR parameters that can be used when interpreting test results and separating normal from abnormal patients. Reviews of large series of tumor patients can help to shed light on the sensitivity and specificity of the various ABR indices.

The Waves I–V interval is generally considered the most robust characteristic of the ABR. Although a number of ABR abnormalities are associated with eighth nerve tumors, a prolonged Waves I–V interval or absence of components beyond Wave I or II is often the most easily interpretable. Because the latency of the Waves I–V interval appears most effective in identifying cerebellopontine angle tumors, it is important to attempt to obtain a clear Wave I using the techniques described above.

In a comparison of ABRs in 32 patients with brainstem lesions and 33 patients with cochlear lesions, the Waves I–V interval was considered the most valuable clinical parameter (Musiek & Lee, 1995). In another series of 75 patients with tumors, the Waves I–V interval was determined to be the most efficient ABR index (Bauch et al., 1996). Combining several parameters may improve sensitivity to brainstem involvement, but also increase the false-positive rate.

Because tumors of the eighth nerve are generally unilateral, comparisons between the two ears can be helpful on a number of different parameters. For example, a patient with a cerebellar astrocytoma showed normal Waves I–V intervals with the only abnormality a prolonged Waves I–III interval in one ear as compared to the other ear (Sostarich, Ferraro, & Karlsen, 1993). Thus, each parameter of the response should be fully considered and entered into the overall clinical interpretation.

In cases where Wave I is not discernible, a combination of measures may prove useful. For example, in a retrospective study of 111 patients with cerebellopontine angle (CPA) tumors and 1370 patients without tumors, Stanton and Cashman (1996) found that, although the Waves I–V interval was the best measure, in instances where that was not available, a combination of Wave V latency and the Wave V interaural latency difference was useful in identifying tumor patients.

5.4.2. Demyelinating and Other Neurological Diseases

The percentage of abnormal ABRs in patients with multiple sclerosis (MS) varies among studies from 0 to 93%, with an average across 16 studies of 61% (Jerger, Oliver, Chmiel, & Rivera, 1986). ABRs in patients with multiple sclerosis may show prolonged interwave latencies, higher amplitude of earlier than later waves in the response, absent waves, and poor replicability (Arnold & Bender, 1983; Chiappa, Harrison, Brooks, & Young, 1980; Jerger et al., 1986; Stockard & Rossiter, 1977; Stockard, Stockard, & Sharbrough, 1980). Chiappa et al. (1980) reported that 32% of 202 patients with multiple sclerosis showed ABRs characterized primarily by abnormal Wave V amplitude and an abnormal Waves III–V interwave latency. Jerger et al. (1986) reported abnormal ABRs in 52% of their 62 patients diagnosed with "definite" multiple sclerosis. By combining the results of ABR with middle ear muscle reflexes, masking level differences, and speech audiometry, identification of auditory abnormalities increased to 90% (Hannley, Jerger, & Rivera, 1983; Jerger et al., 1986).

Stockard et al. (1980) reported that increased interwave latency was diagnostically more definitive than amplitude. Controversy exists over whether increases in stimulus rate can enhance latency changes in patients with multiple sclerosis

(Chiappa et al., 1980; Robinson & Rudge, 1977). Treatment and periods of remission in multiple sclerosis may be reflected by changes in the characteristics of the ABR (Chiappa et al., 1980; Robinson & Rudge, 1977; Stockard & Rossiter, 1977). Abnormal ABR, absent MEMRs, and reduced speech recognition have also been associated with sudden-onset hearing loss related to multiple sclerosis (Stach & Delgado-Vilches, 1993).

Abnormal ABRs have been reported in patients with Parkinson's disease (Gawal, Das, Vincent, & Rose, 1981), with global cerebral insults (Sanders, Smirga, McCullough, & Duncan, 1981), and in patients who are comatose as a result of blunt head trauma (Seales, Rossiter, & Weinstein, 1979). Asymmetric ABRs have been reported in cases of albinism (Chédiak-Higashi syndrome) where there is a suspected misrouting of auditory pathways (Creel, Boxer, & Fauci, 1983). Neurological evaluation using the ABR also has application in pediatric neurological diseases and therefore should not be limited to the adult population (Hecox, Cone, & Blaw, 1981).

Abnormal ABRs occurred in 6 of 60 children tested who had recovered from bacterial meningitis (Özdamar & Kraus, 1983). Generally, the children with abnormal ABRs also showed other complications, and seizures, respiratory distress, and hydrocephaly were not uncommon. The remaining patients either were normal audiologically and neurologically or had ABRs consistent with peripheral hearing loss.

5.4.3. Other Neural Disorders Affecting the ABR

5.4.3.1. Auditory Neuropathy

Recently, a group of patients has been described who demonstrate normal otoacoustic emissions and absent or grossly abnormal ABRs, having what has been termed an auditory neuropathy (Berlin et al., 1993; Starr et al., 1996). Normal otoacoustic emissions suggest normal outer hair cell function while the abnormal ABRs suggest a neural disorder, which, in the absence of a space-occupying lesion or disorder such as multiple sclerosis, distinguishes auditory neuropathy from these other types of neurological conditions. Some patients with auditory neuropathy demonstrate timing problems (Starr et al., 1991), which are suggestive of a disturbance in neural synchrony.

Specific diagnostic measures that can help to distinguish cochlear from neural function include MEMRs, otoacoustic emissions, ECochG, and ABR. Patients with auditory neuropathy demonstrate a disruption of function at the level of the inner hair cell and/or auditory nerve in the presence of normal outer hair cell function. Most patients with auditory neuropathy show bilateral symptoms, al-

Table 5-3. Test findings in patients with auditory neuropathy.

Measurement	Finding
Pure-tone thresholds	Variable (normal to severe)
Tympanograms	Normal (if no middle ear pathology)
Middle ear muscle reflexes	
Ipsilateral	Absent
Contralateral	Absent
Nonacoustic	Present
Otoacoustic emissions	Normal
Cochlear microphonic	Present
Auditory brainstem response	Absent or abnormal
Masking level differences	Absent
Otoacoustic emission suppression	Absent

though function may be asymmetric between ears and a few cases of unilateral auditory neuropathy have been documented.

Some early reports documented abnormal ABRs in patients who later were found to have normal cochlear function (Kraus, Özdamar, Stein, & Reed, 1984; Worthington & Peters, 1980). These patients were studied before otoacoustic emissions were in use clinically. With the availability of otoacoustic emissions and measurement of the cochlear microphonic, investigators can examine cochlear function, specifically outer hair cell function, in patients who have no ABRs (e.g., Berlin et al., 1993; Berlin, Hood, Hurley, & Wen, 1994; Gorga, Stelmachowicz, Barlow, & Brookhouser, 1995; Kaga et al., 1996; Starr et al., 1991).

Clinical findings in patients with an auditory neuropathy show variable pure-tone thresholds, ranging from normal sensitivity to severe or profound hearing loss. MEMR responses to acoustic stimuli are absent. Otoacoustic emissions, in the absence of any middle ear pathology, are normal and sometimes remarkably larger than normally observed. ABRs are consistently abnormal and, in many patients, *no* synchronous neural response to brief stimuli such as clicks is present. Masking level differences (MLD) are abnormal with patients generally showing no masking level difference. Speech recognition is quite variable though generally much poorer than expected based on pure-tone thresholds (based on word recognition norms; Yellin, Jerger, & Fifer, 1989). Table 5–3 summarizes findings in patients with an auditory neuropathy.

The use of a test battery approach that includes both the ABR and otoacoustic emissions is critical in identifying these patients. Normal outer hair cell function is evidenced by the presence of otoacoustic emissions and cochlear microphonics. Abnormal neural function is reflected by abnormal ABRs and MEMRs. In patients with poor otoacoustic emissions, it may be possible to record cochlear microphonic responses. Ipsilateral masking can be used to distinguish the cochlear microphonic from a neural response because masking will reduce the amplitude of the ABR, more readily the cochlear microphonic.

The classification of auditory neuropathy most likely describes several different specific sites of abnormality, all of which result in the clinical observation of normal outer hair cell responses accompanied by poor neural responses. Some patients, both children and adults, have no known etiology and no other identified neurological abnormalities. In other patients, the auditory findings may be associated with other peripheral neuropathies. Examples are patients with hereditary motor sensory neuropathy (HMSN; Charcot-Marie-Tooth disease) or Friedreich's ataxia, which affect the motor periphery (see Case Study 16). Infants with neonatal abnormalities, including hyperbilirubinemia, have been reported with auditory neuropathy (Deltenre, Mansbach, Bozet, Clercx, & Hecox, 1997; Stein et al., 1996). There are also cases where a genetic basis is suspected due to multiple affected family members.

Auditory neuropathies have been reported in infants, children, and adults. Proper recording and interpretation of the ABR in infants and children are particularly important in pediatric cases, because responses that appear on the surface to be a neural response are, in fact, cochlear responses that may span a time period of 5 to 6 ms (Berlin et al., 1998). Cochlear and neural responses can be distinguished by reversing the polarity of the stimulus. A cochlear microphonic response will invert with polarity reversal whereas a neural response will not, possibly showing only a slight latency shift. Use of alternating-polarity stimuli (which is not recommended) will obliterate the cochlear response. Use of rapid recording techniques such as maximum length sequences also results in reduced ability to see the cochlear response (Berlin et al., 1998). A case study of an infant with an auditory neuropathy is presented in Case Study 17 in Chapter 8.

Management of patients with an auditory neuropathy requires special considerations because standard approaches may not be of value. Standard amplification does not seem to benefit most individuals with auditory neuropathy. Some patients benefit from FM (frequency modulation) devices, most likely due to improved signal-to-noise ratios that provide a clearer signal to a system that cannot cope with interference. Also, in the cases of infants and children, some visual system, such as Cued Speech or a manual communication system that follows the grammatical structure of the patient's primary language, may be helpful in facilitating language development. It is currently unknown whether electrical stimulation, such as through a cochlear implant, would be beneficial. Further confounding management issues related to infants and children with auditory neuropathy are reports that *some* of these young patients appear to be "outgrowing" the neuropathy and developing some auditory responses and skills (Berlin et al., 1998; Stein et al., 1996). Although the probability of this is simply not known at present, the importance of management for all children with auditory neuropathy lies in facilitating development of language and communication skills.

The mechanisms of auditory neuropathy presently are unclear, and it is most likely that several mechanisms and types of auditory neuropathy exist. There are, based on the auditory and neurological data, several possibilities. Auditory neuropathy also may have several etiologies. The mechanical transduction or other functional characteristics of the inner hair cells could be abnormal, the synaptic juncture between the inner hair cells and the cochlear branch of the vestibulo-cochlear (eighth) nerve could be affected, or the axons or cell bodies of the eighth nerve itself could be the site.

Despite the diversity of possible etiologies, the auditory findings are quite uniform and the ABR plays a key role in identifying those patients with auditory neuropathy. Of the test results summarized in Table 5–3, the combination of normal otoacoustic emissions and abnormal or absent ABR represents a key combination in identification. The role of the various auditory measures and the outcomes in adults and infants are demonstrated in Case Studies 16 and 17, respectively.

5.4.3.2. Fourth Ventricle Hydroencephaly

The ABR is often abnormal in cases of fourth ventricle hydroencephaly (Kraus, Özdamar, Heydemann, Stein, & Reed, 1984; Stach, Wolf, & Bland, 1995). ABR and clinical findings were examined in 40 patients with confirmed hydrocephalus by Kraus, Özdamar, Heydemann, et al. (1984). ABRs were abnormal in 88% of the patients and ABR thresholds were elevated or absent in 70% of the patients. In these cases, as in other patients where the brainstem region is specifically affected, otoacoustic emissions and other auditory measures can be particularly helpful in determining cochlear function and the site of the disorder.

5.4.3.3. Vascular Abnormalities

Prolonged ABR latencies have been reported in patients with type I (insulin-dependent) diabetes (Virtaniemi, Laasko, Karja, Nuutinen, & Karjalainen, 1993). Wave V latencies and Waves I–V intervals were prolonged in a series of 53 diabetic patients, which were most likely related to the long duration of the diabetes and microvascular complications associated with the disease.

5.4.4. Head Injury

The ABR has been used in patients with severe head injury. This has been particularly valuable because recovery of severely head-injured patients depends to a large extent on damage to brainstem areas. While auditory areas would of course need to be affected to result in abnormalities on an ABR, reports have shown that patients with ABRs where all waves are preserved are more likely to have a favorable outcome than patients with no ABR or absence of components (Mjøen, Nordby, & Torvik, 1983; Ottaviani, Almadori, Calderazzo, Frenguelli, & Paludetti, 1986). Although the outcome is not accurately predicted in 100% of the cases, the ABR results do show some tendencies and thus may contribute information of use in viewing overall prognosis.

5.4.5. Coma and Brain Death

The ABR has been applied with varying degrees of success in cases of coma and in the definition of brain death (Hall & Mackey-Hargadine, 1984) and in determination of the etiology and reversibility of coma (Stockard et al., 1980). The presence of a solitary Wave I is reported in brain death and can be useful in the evaluation of patients with isoelectric EEGs (Starr, 1977; Starr & Hamilton, 1976).

5.5. USE OF THE ABR IN INTRAOPERATIVE AND INTENSIVE CARE UNIT MONITORING

The ABR is used to monitor neural function during removal of tumors of the auditory nerve. Because of differences in the circumstances under which the ABR is performed, there are numerous issues not encountered in the clinic that must be considered when applying ABR testing successfully in the operating room.

One of the greatest technical problems to overcome in ABR monitoring in the operating room is a noisy environment, both electrically and acoustically. Electrical interference can present the most challenging obstacles, and planning and work with operating room personnel can be helpful in addressing some of these problems. Use of some type of insert earphone, either the ER-3 earphones or custom-made earmolds, is mandatory because the position of the patient's head may change after the earphone is placed without opportunity to observe the position of the earphone once it is set in place.

A baseline response should be obtained for both ears after the patient is prepared but before the procedure begins. This will serve as the standard for comparison throughout the procedure. Rapid recording with frequently updated responses is recommended. Changes in the ABR generally occur throughout critical portions of the procedure, and the audiologist or technician should compare responses online throughout the surgical procedure and store waveforms for later comparison. Whenever significant changes are observed, the surgeon should be informed immediately so that he or she can consider appropriate measures to take.

Recommendation is made that both ears be monitored, with the noninvolved ear serving as an ongoing reference. Thus, changes in body temperature during the procedure and other factors that affect the patient as a whole can be accounted for by comparing the response from the noninvolved ear to that from the operated side.

Another useful procedure is to monitor action potentials directly from the auditory nerve in a near-field recording technique where an electrode is secured adjacent to the cochlear nerve (e.g., Roberson, Senne, Brackmann, Hitselberger, & Saunders, 1996; Wazen, 1994). Standard techniques can be used with click stimuli and, because recordings are obtained in the near field, waveforms are high in amplitude relative to the background noise and responses can be observed in seconds rather than the minutes required for far-field averaging. Direct eighth nerve recordings thus allow nearly real-time recording of responses and observation of immediate changes in waveform amplitude and/or latency during the surgical procedure. Whereas some investigators report superiority of this method over the surface-recorded ABR, others report that either direct recording or ABR result in similar success in preserving hearing (Cohen, Lewis, & Ransohoff, 1993).

In a series of 144 cases of acoustic neuroma removal reported by Harner, Harper, Beatty, Litchy, and Ebersold (1996), factors of importance included tumor size, preoperative auditory function, and preoperative presence of Wave V. In their experience, preservation of hearing was rare in tumors greater than 2.5 cm and preserving Wave V during surgery did not guarantee preservation of hearing postoperatively. However, loss of Wave V during surgery did not always result in loss of hearing postoperatively.

In another retrospective study of 93 patients who underwent acoustic neuroma removal via the middle fossa approach, useful hearing was preserved in 58% of patients and hearing was preserved to near preoperative levels in 45% of patients (Dornhoffer, Helms, & Hoehmann, 1995). In this study, the potential for hearing preservation appeared inversely related to the size of the tumor. This is consistent with the retrospective study of 161 patients by Cohen et al. (1993), who also reported that origin from the superior vestibular nerve is a favorable prognostic indicator. Conversely, other studies have not found tumor size predictive of postoperative outcome (Aoyagi et al., 1994).

Another important issue is the long-term stability of hearing following acoustic neuroma surgery. In a follow-up study, 17 patients with successful preservation of hearing immediately after retrosigmoid approach surgery were reevaluated at 1.5 to 8 years after surgery (Tucci, Telian, Kileny, Hoff, & Kemick, 1994). Although some patients showed decreases in pure-tone sensitivity or speech recognition, others showed increases, and overall all patients maintained usable hearing.

Table 5–4. Strengths and limitations of the ABR in neurological applications.

Strengths	Limitations
Sensitive to space-occupying lesions and neural pathway integrity	Not sensitive to central nervous system disorders above the brainstem
High abnormal rate in patients with eighth nerve tumors	Affected by peripheral hearing loss
Noninvasive	May miss small eighth nerve tumors
Normal response well-defined	Some subjectivity in marking waveforms
Good normal response reliability	

5.6. STRENGTHS AND LIMITATIONS OF THE ABR IN NEUROLOGICAL APPLICATIONS

The ABR provides a powerful clinical method to evaluate the neural integrity of the eighth nerve and auditory brainstem pathways. Understanding both the strengths and limitations enhances the clinician's ability to appropriately use the ABR in patients with suspected neurological disorders (see Table 5–4).

5.6.1. Strengths of the ABR

The ABR provides a noninvasive method of evaluating the integrity of the auditory nerve and brainstem pathways. It represents neural activity and thus provides information about neural function of the lower auditory system. The ABR is particularly useful in patients without radiologically identifiable lesions who have functional abnormalities of the peripheral auditory pathways such as an auditory neuropathy.

High sensitivity of the ABR is reported in identifying tumors of the auditory nerve and brainstem, though radiological techniques (i.e., MRI with gadolinium contrast) may be able to identify some very small tumors where the ABR may not (e.g., Naessens, Gordts, Clement, & Buisseret, 1996). The ABR may be of particular use in settings where MRI is not available and may be recommended to select priority patients for MRI in situations where waiting lists are long (Ferguson et al., 1996).

The latencies of the waves in the normal ABR are highly replicable, providing a powerful basis for judging abnormality. Predictable changes occur with changes in intensity, and some components of the response are observed at levels within

15 to 20 dB of behavioral threshold. With some limitations, the ABR provides information about peripheral hearing and can be used to distinguish among different types of hearing loss.

5.6.2. Limitations of the ABR in Neurological Applications

Perhaps one of the greatest limitations and frustrations in using the ABR occurs in the evaluation of patients with substantial peripheral hearing loss. The effectiveness of the stimulus is decreased by peripheral hearing loss, which impairs clear definition of waveforms and clouds the interpretation of differences between ears. In cases of severe high-frequency hearing loss, it may be impossible to obtain an ABR. However, the presence of a severe or even total audiometric loss should not rule out the use of ABR because normal Waves I and II are seen occasionally with patients who have no audiometric response.

The ABR is not sensitive to all central nervous system disorders. The test does not evaluate the integrity of the nervous system rostral to (above) the brainstem, so cortical auditory deafness cannot be ruled out on the basis of a normal ABR (Hood, Berlin, & Allen, 1994).

In waveform examination there is no clearly defined method for latency determination or quantification of morphology and replicability. Thus, latency determination is dependent on the particular point on a waveform that is chosen by the examiner as the peak (Lazor & Melnick, 1984). Wave V is often difficult to identify because Waves IV and V fuse together in ipsilateral recordings. In rounded waveforms either the peak of the wave or the change in slope from the peak to the following negative trough is used as a latency indicator. We often determine absolute waveform latency for Wave V by starting at V' (the following negative trough) and tracing backward to the point where there is a change in the slope.

Knowledge of the status of peripheral hearing is critical to the management of cases. In patients where no Wave I is present and Wave V is delayed, knowledge of bone-conduction sensitivity and the presence of an air-bone gap is useful because both eighth nerve disorders and conductive losses can result in a delayed Wave V. It is particularly important to rule out the presence of a conductive and/or severe hearing loss when evaluating comatose patients because hearing loss may obliterate a response.

5.7. TECHNICAL ERRORS

Some of the limitations of the ABR are related to technical problems that result from improper test set-up or procedures. Table 5–5 lists considerations related to response acquisition and interpretation.

Table 5-5. Considerations in neurological applications related to response acquisition and interpretation.

Procedure	Consideration

Response acquisition:	1. Electrode impedance low and balanced
	2. Electrodes correctly connected
	3. Earphones in place
	4. Patient relaxed
	5. Proper stimulus
	   • type
	   • intensity
	   • polarity
	   • presentation rate
	   • ear stimulated
	6. Recording
	   • time window
	   • filter band
	   • amplification
	7. Check for ear canal collapse or use insert earphones

Response interpretation:	1. Replicability 2. Latency, amplitude 3. Rate effect 4. Response symmetry between ears 5. Peripheral hearing loss considered 6. Cross-check results with middle ear status, MEMR thresholds, OAE results, other tests.

Note: MEMR = middle ear muscle reflex; OAE = otoacoustic emissions.

Careful control of stimulus intensity and stimulus delivery is necessary to ensure appropriate data for analysis of waveform latencies and of thresholds of responses. Ear canal collapse (Ventry, Chaiklin, & Boyle, 1962) or earphone slippage can reduce signal intensity at the ear without the examiner's knowledge. Improperly calibrated stimuli can also compromise test accuracy.

Improper subject preparation can result in noisy or difficult to interpret recordings. Poor electrode impedance or dissimilar impedances among electrodes may yield poorly defined, difficult to interpret responses. Subjects who are very tense, not advised of the need to relax, or placed in an uncomfortable position or environment may produce excessive muscle artifact.

Technical errors in equipment setup, such as inappropriate connection of the electrodes or amplification of the biological signal, may result in erroneous recordings. The artifact rejection system may be set at a rejection level so sensitive that the peaks of the response are cut off if they exceed the artifact rejection level. In testing infants and young children who may be neurologically immature and/

or have hearing loss, it is possible to miss a prolonged response (e.g., in the 10- to 15-ms time window) if too short of a time window (e.g., 10 ms) is used.

5.8. CROSS-CHECK AMONG TESTS

The use of a test battery approach, that is, a number of measures that are sensitive to the abnormality in question, can strengthen findings. The ABR correlates well with results of other behavioral and physiological tests and thus supports test battery and cross-check principles. Use of a single measure often will result in ambiguous findings, whereas combinations of tests can reduce this ambiguity.

The ABR, MEMRs, and speech audiometry (word recognition in noise, synthetic sentence identification with competing message), if used singly in the evaluation of auditory nerve or brainstem lesions, may result in some ambiguity due to middle ear and cochlear factors (Jerger, Neely, & Jerger, 1980). MEMRs are modified by both middle ear and cochlear disorders, speech recognition is influenced by cochlear abnormalities, and the ABR can be modified by disorders at every level of the auditory system through the brainstem. Pairing results with the audiogram reduces ambiguity and combining ABR, MEMR, and speech recognition creates a test battery that can more clearly identify eighth nerve/brainstem lesions.

Other measures, including interaural timing or phase processing procedures, such as the masking level difference, are also sensitive to auditory brainstem lesions (e.g., Musiek, Gollegy, Kibbe, & Verkest, 1988). The combination of an abnormal ABR with abnormal CT or MRI scans and abnormal MEMR thresholds further strengthens the identification of patients with occult neurological disease affecting the auditory system. These measures and principles will be further reviewed in the discussions of the case studies presented in Chapter 8.

6

Clinical Application of the ABR in Estimating Hearing Sensitivity

Auditory evoked potentials, when used and interpreted properly, provide a powerful method of obtaining reliable estimates of auditory sensitivity in infants, young children, and other individuals who cannot or will not provide reliable results on behavioral hearing tests. Indeed, Hallowell Davis' pioneering work with the cortical potentials was, in part, directed toward the development of a technique to assess auditory function without the need for patient participation. Evoked potentials from the cochlea to the cortex have been studied as possible methods to assess hearing. Some responses work well; some have proved less than ideal.

Although the auditory brainstem response (ABR) is not a test of hearing sensitivity per se, the information obtained can be useful in estimating hearing sensitivity. This chapter will discuss various types of frequency-specific stimuli, the use of bone-conducted stimuli, procedures used for this type of evaluation, and the relationship between evoked potential thresholds and behavioral thresholds.

6.1. A BRIEF HISTORICAL PERSPECTIVE

If the goal of hearing testing is to determine peripheral hearing sensitivity, then measurement of responses directly from the cochlea would seem ideal. In fact, electrocochleography (ECochG) proved a very useful technique in the 1960s and 1970s. However, the somewhat invasive nature of transtympanic or eardrum recording sites limited its widespread clinical application. Cortical responses and middle latency responses, studied in the 1950s and 1960s, proved useful but required that the subject be awake, cooperative, and alert during testing. These factors limited applications in infants and children, the population most needing an objective "hearing test" method. The relative ease of recording the ABR and its resistance to the effects of sleep and sedation have facilitated its widespread use in hearing assessment of infants, children, and, to a lesser extent, adults.

6.2. WHAT AUDITORY EVOKED POTENTIALS TEST

Although the ABR has proved useful in estimating hearing sensitivity, it is important to remember that the ABR is *not* a test of hearing! The ABR and other evoked potentials test neural synchrony, that is, the ability of the central nervous system to respond to external stimulation in a synchronous manner. This synchronous neural response results from the firing of a large group of neurons at the same time.

REMEMBER:
The auditory brainstem response is NOT a hearing test.

When the central nervous system is functioning normally, neural responses can be used to record evoked potentials to stimuli presented at various intensity levels. Thus, the clinician can find the lowest intensity level where the neural response is elicited and relate that to a threshold for hearing. ABRs can be obtained at intensities close to behavioral thresholds if a sufficient number of responses (on the order of 10,000) are averaged to adequately reduce the background physiological noise (Elberling & Don, 1987). In routine clinical procedures where fewer averages are used, responses can generally be obtained near, but not at, behavioral thresholds.

6.3. WHEN TO USE THE ABR TO ESTIMATE AUDITORY FUNCTION

The ABR is best used when the clinician desires a noninvasive, safe approach to assess auditory function in infants, children, and adults who cannot participate in voluntary audiometry. Evoked potentials are especially useful when one wishes to know the sensitivity of each cochlea separately, to compare responses by air conduction and bone conduction with or without masking, and to estimate auditory function in frequency-specific ranges. Because the ABR is a test of the neural system, insight into the integrity of the neural pathways from the eighth nerve through portions of the brainstem can also be obtained. Evoked potentials should not be used in lieu of a behavioral audiogram in patients who can provide reliable behavioral responses; an ultimate goal in all patients should be to obtain behavioral responses. In infants and young children, behavioral responses may be obtained at a later time, but, in the meantime, appropriate management can begin based on ABR results.

6.4. CLICKS VERSUS FREQUENCY-SPECIFIC STIMULI

A 100-microsecond electrical pulse, impressed on a standard earphone, generates a broadband signal (click) whose primary frequency emphasis is determined by the resonant frequency of the transducer. With the use of standard TDH-39 or TDH-49 supra-aural earphones or of ER-3 insert earphones, the maximum energy peaks are in the frequency region between 1000 and 4000 Hz (H. Davis, 1976; H. Davis & Hirsh, 1979; Don, Eggermont, & Brackmann, 1979). The greatest agreement with pure-tone thresholds is in the 2000 to 4000 Hz frequency range (Bauch & Olsen, 1986, 1987). Thus a click, though a broadband stimulus, is nonetheless somewhat frequency specific based primarily on the frequency response of the earphones.

When using frequency-specific stimuli there is a trade-off between frequency specificity and neural synchrony. The acoustic principle underlying this trade-off involves the relationship between the duration of a stimulus and its frequency

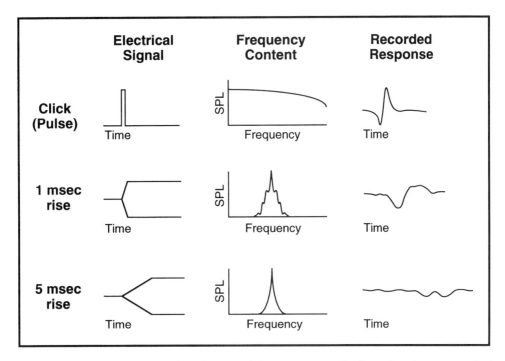

Figure 6-1. Comparison of stimulus onset, frequency content, and surface-recorded responses for a click, a toneburst with a 1-ms rise time, and a toneburst with a 5-ms rise time.

content (see Figure 6–1). The longer the duration of a stimulus, the more frequency specific the stimulus will be. An example of a very frequency-specific stimulus (i.e., a single frequency) is a pure tone, which has a long rise time and duration. Because of their long onset, single pure tones are not efficient in eliciting an ABR. In contrast, a click, which is abrupt in onset and brief in duration, is better able to elicit a synchronous neural response but is not very frequency specific.

If we could place an electrode directly on a nerve fiber responsive to a certain frequency, then it might be possible to asses the response of that nerve fiber using a pure-tone stimulus. However, because the ABR uses a far-field recording method (i.e., on the surface of the scalp), we must activate a large number of neurons at precisely the same moment in order to "see" a response.

Again, basic acoustic principles dictate that the more abrupt the acoustic onset of a stimulus, the more frequencies that stimulus contains. Stimulating a broad region of the cochlear partition all at once will activate a large number of neurons simultaneously, resulting in a synchronous neural discharge (in a normal system). The more synchronous the neural discharge, the better the resulting ABR, but the poorer the frequency specificity. When interpreting results, it is important to remember that the use of tonebursts results in stimulation of the cochlea at frequency regions surrounding the target frequency as well as at the desired frequency. Thus, tonebursts are more frequency specific than clicks, but not as frequency specific as pure tones.

6.5. TYPES OF FREQUENCY-SPECIFIC STIMULI

Several types of stimuli and recording methods have been proposed to provide information for narrower frequency regions (see Table 6–1). Some alternative stimuli and methods include tonebursts, filtered clicks, tonebursts and clicks mixed with various types of noise, and high-pass masking of clicks. Each type of stimulus appears to have advantages and limitations, and stimulus selection is dependent on the desired frequency specificity, the type of response being recorded, the amount of time available for testing, and the equipment available. Because tonebursts are the most commonly used type of frequency specific stimuli in ABR testing, much of the information to follow will focus on the use of tonebursts.

6.5.1. Tonebursts

In a study designed to find the "best compromise" stimulus that would maximize both frequency specificity and neural synchrony, H. Davis, Hirsh, Turpin, and Peacock (1985) recommended a toneburst with two cycles (or periods) of rise time, a one-cycle plateau, and two cycles of decay (sometimes referred to as a 2-1-2 envelope). To convert this information to actual stimulus duration in units of time, one must recall information about the physical characteristics of sine waves in relation to frequency and duration.

It takes 1 ms for a 1000-Hz tone to complete one cycle (or period).[1] A 500-Hz tone, which is lower in frequency, takes more time to complete one cycle (1000 ms/500 = 2 ms per cycle). Conversely, a 2000-Hz tone takes less time to complete a cycle (1000 ms/2000 = 0.5 ms). See Table 6–2 for a comparison of frequency, single cycle durations, and recommended toneburst durations.

Because one period of a 500-Hz tone is 2 ms in duration, a 500-Hz toneburst derived according to the recommendations of H. Davis et al. (1985) would have an envelope of 4 ms of rise time, a 2-ms plateau, and 4 ms of decay time. More recently, in many practices the plateau has been dropped because it contributes little to frequency specificity. Thus, a 2-0-2 envelope is often used where, for a

---

[1] If one recalls that the earlier terminology for the term *Hz* was *cycles per second* (or cps), then it is fairly straightforward to determine that a 1000-Hz or 1000-cps stimulus has 1000 cycles per second. There are 1000 ms in 1 s, so 1 cycle or 1/1000 of 1000 cps would take 1 ms to complete.

Table 6-1. Types of frequency-specific stimuli for auditory evoked potential testing.

Filtered clicks

Clicks with high-pass noise

Tonebursts

Tonebursts with high-pass noise

Tonebursts in notched noise

Amplitude-modulated (AM) tones

Frequency-modulated (FM) tones

Table 6-2. Parameters for tonebursts at different frequencies using 2-0-2 cycle envelopes.

Center Frequency (Hz)	Duration of a Single Cycle (ms)	Duration of a 2-0-2 Envelope (Rise–Plateau–Fall)	Total Stimulus Duration (ms)
250	4	8 ms–0 ms–8 ms	16
500	2	4 ms–0 ms–4 ms	8
1000	1	2 ms–0 ms–2 ms	4
2000	.5	1 ms–0 ms–1 ms	2
4000	.25	.5 ms–0 ms–.5 ms	1
8000	.125	.25 ms–0 ms–.25 ms	.5

500 Hz toneburst, the rise and fall times would be 4 ms each for a total stimulus duration of 8 ms.

Changes in envelope characteristics affect the spectrum of the stimulus, the physical intensity of the stimulus, and the loudness due to durational changes and temporal integration. The latency of the response is also affected in that longer rise times result in increased latency. By holding the number of periods in the stimulus constant across different frequencies, the power spectrum can be held constant (H. Davis, Hirsh, & Turpin, 1983).

In addition, the onset and offset (envelope) characteristics of the stimulus also affect the spectral or frequency characteristics of the stimulus. A linear rise and fall of energy is characterized by an abrupt change from no stimulus to the rise of energy and a sharp change when the plateau is reached (see Figure 6–2). If an envelope is used that has a more gradual onset and offset function, such as a cosine-squared, Blackmann, or Hanning function, then there is less spectral spread of energy into other frequency ranges. Thus, when given the choice, it

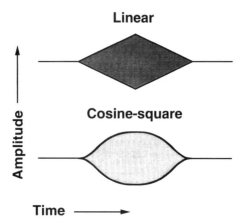

Figure 6-2. Comparison of linear and cosine-square envelopes.

may be desirable to use other than a linear envelope to maintain as much frequency specificity in the stimulus as possible.

6.5.2. Stimulus Polarity Effects With Tonebursts

The choice of stimulus polarity is particularity important when using toneburst stimuli. When the polarity of a toneburst stimulus is reversed, latency shifts in the peak of the response are observed. Whereas higher frequency tonebursts (e.g., 2000 or 3000 Hz) show little or no latency shift with polarity reversals (similar to clicks), tonebursts centered at lower frequencies, such as 250 or 500 Hz, can show large latency shifts that can degrade the waveform and even be out of phase with responses to stimuli of the opposite polarity (Gorga, Kaminski, & Beauchaine, 1991; Orlando & Folsom, 1995). As shown in Figure 6–3, Wave V shows a marked latency shift with polarity changes for 500-Hz tonebursts and is difficult to discern with alternating polarity tonebursts. A similar effect is not seen for 3000-Hz tonebursts. Thus, although it may seem intuitively desirable to use alternating polarity tonebursts to minimize stimulus artifact, in fact the use of alternating tonebursts for lower frequencies can be detrimental to response quality.

6.5.3. High-Frequency Tonebursts

Although the focus of the use of the ABR for evaluation of hearing sensitivity is generally directed toward quantifying hearing sensitivity in lower frequency regions, high-frequency tonebursts are also useful in some circumstances. Fausti and colleagues have studied the generation and recording of ABRs using high-frequency tonebursts in some detail, with particular application to monitoring

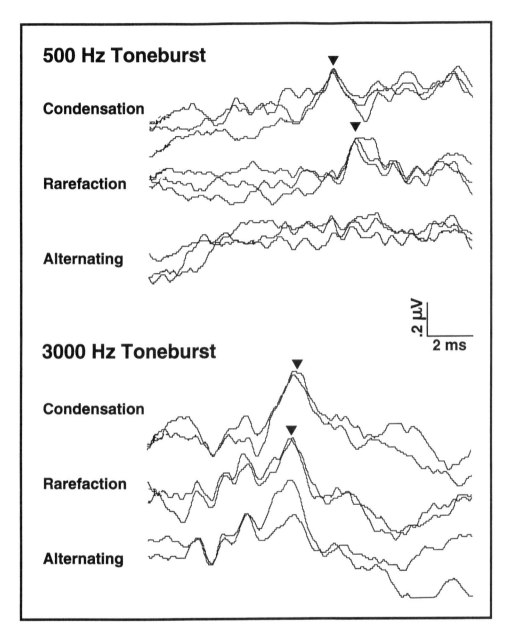

Figure 6–3. ABRs obtained with tonebursts centered at 500 Hz (*top*) and 3000 Hz (*bottom*). Responses obtained with 500-Hz tonebursts show latency shifts between condensation and rarefaction polarities and significantly reduced responses when alternating-polarity tonebursts are used. Only slight latency shifts are present with 3000-Hz tonebursts, resulting in less amplitude reduction with alternating-polarity stimuli.

the effects of ototoxic medications. ABR testing with high-frequency tonebursts generally is directed toward patients who are ill, unresponsive, or otherwise difficult to test behaviorally. A five-frequency range of tonebursts centered at 8000

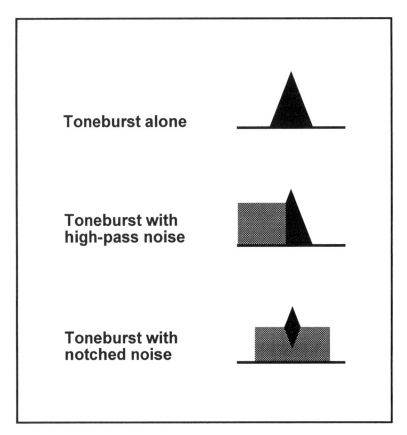

Figure 6–4. Schematic representation of a toneburst alone, a toneburst with high-pass noise, and a toneburst in notched noise. Black triangle represents a toneburst; gray rectangle represents noise.

to 14,000 Hz has been shown to be reliable for stimuli presented sequentially at each single frequency and in multiple-frequency sets (Fausti, Mitchell, Frey, Henry, & O'Connor, 1994). High-frequency toneburst ABRs have been shown to identify changes in sensitivity in as many as 93% of patients monitored for ototoxic effects (Fausti, Frey, Henry, Olson, & Schaffer, 1993). Normal values for latency as a function of intensity have been generated for normal-hearing subjects as well as individuals with sensory hearing loss (Fausti, Olsen, Frey, Henry, & Schaffer, 1993; Fausti et al., 1995).

6.5.4. Masking Noise With Clicks and Tonebursts

Several methods involving masking of clicks and tonebursts have been used in an effort to obtain greater control over the frequency content of the stimulus. A schematic of some of these stimulus paradigms is shown in Figure 6–4.

6.5.5. High-Pass Masking of Clicks

In a method pioneered by Teas, Eldredge, and Davis (1962), the cutoff frequency of a high-pass masker is progressively decreased and ABRs are obtained for each of the cutoff frequencies. Then the click-elicited ABRs at adjacent masker cutoff frequencies are subtracted from each other, resulting in a series of "derived responses" representing the presence of neural activity in different frequency bands (Don & Eggermont, 1978; Parker & Thornton, 1978a, 1978b). Because the high-pass noise appears to desynchronize neural output in the frequency regions of the masker noise, the remaining response represents neural activity in frequency regions below that of the noise cutoff frequency.

The derived band method allows separation of frequency-specific wave components and has been shown to be useful in audiogram reconstruction (Don et al., 1979). This method provides control over the frequency region being assessed, although it requires collection of a large number of responses (which can be time consuming), the capability to generate high-pass masking noise at various cutoff frequencies, presentation of the noise and click through the same transducer, and both storage and subtraction capability in the equipment.

6.5.6. High-Pass Masking and Tonebursts

Another method uses tonebursts presented in the presence of a high-pass masker (Kileny, 1981). By presenting stimuli simultaneously with a masker, the higher frequency regions of the cochlea are masked with the obtained responses representing activity from lower frequency regions of the cochlea. Kileny (1981) compared responses to low-frequency tonebursts with and without a high-pass masker and found that the latency of the masked tonebursts was longer than that of the unmasked toneburst, suggesting that the presence of the masker resulted in a shift of the response to a lower frequency region.

6.5.7. Tonebursts in Notched Noise

Presentation of tonebursts and clicks in notched noise has been suggested as a modification of the derived method (Picton et al., 1979; Pratt & Bleich, 1982). The notched-noise method is considered more efficient because multiple recordings and subtraction of waveforms for each response are unnecessary. The utility of this method has been demonstrated, particularly for tonal stimuli, although additional special equipment may be necessary to filter the noise, and the masker level is critical.

Notched noise is a noise in which less noise is generated in a specific range of frequencies, resulting in the appearance of the notch in the noise in the frequency region of the stimulus (see Figure 6–4). The notched noise is used to restrict the responsiveness of the cochlear partition to frequencies within the region of the notch, which is set at the frequency range of interest. An advantage of using tonal stimuli rather than clicks is the lower intensity of the masker noise necessary to mask energy outside of the notch. This allows a greater concentration of stimulus energy around the frequency of interest.

The use of notched noise with high-intensity stimuli does not alter the latency of high-frequency tones but does reduce response amplitude. For high-intensity stimuli centered at 500 and 1000 Hz, notched noise affects both amplitude and latency of the response. The change in latency is most likely due to the spectral spread of energy of tonebursts at higher intensities, which can be limited with the notched noise. Comparisons of tonebursts without noise, tonebursts in notched noise, and tonebursts in broadband noise suggest that the use of noise may be more important for higher intensity tonebursts than when testing at lower intensities (e.g., Beattie & Kennedy, 1992). Thus, the use of notched noise at lower intensities (on the order of 40 to 50 dB nHL) for all frequencies does not seem as critical because less spread of spectral energy occurs (e.g., Beattie, Thielen, & Franzone, 1994; Stapells, Picton, Perez-Abalo, Read, & Smith, 1985).

When thresholds obtained using tonebursts in notched noise are compared to behavioral thresholds, differences between thresholds obtained using the two methods decrease as frequency increases in normal-hearing subjects and hearing-impaired patients (Beattie, Garcia, & Johnson, 1996; Sininger & Abdala, 1998; Stapells, Gravel, & Martin, 1995; Stapells, Picton, Durieux-Smith, Edwards, & Moran, 1990). Threshold differences generally are in the range of 20 dB for lower frequencies (500 and 1000 Hz) and 10 dB for higher frequencies (2000 and 4000 Hz), although some studies have shown agreement of approximately 10 dB in the lower frequencies as well.

6.6. PROCEDURES IN USING THE ABR TO ESTIMATE HEARING SENSITIVITY

Estimates of hearing sensitivity can be obtained from ABR data by progressively decreasing the intensity of the stimulus (click or toneburst) until no response is discernible. Because Wave V remains at lower intensities, the approach often used is to begin at levels well above the anticipated threshold (based on the case history or other audiometric testing) and then decrease intensity by steps of 10 to 20 dB while following the progressive increase in Wave V latency. An ABR test battery that includes recordings for three different stimuli is described for infants, children, and adults.

Table 6–3. Auditory brainstem response test stimuli and what they evaluate.

Stimulus	What Is Evaluated
Air-conduction clicks	Higher frequencies
	External ear, middle ear, cochlea, eighth nerve, brainstem
500-Hz tonebursts	Lower frequencies
	External ear, middle ear, cochlea, eighth nerve, brainstem
Bone-conduction clicks	Higher frequencies
	Cochlea, eighth nerve, brainstem

Table 6–4. Three-part test protocol for the estimation of hearing sensitivity in infants and young children.

Stimulus/Target	Response
Air conduction (higher frequencies)	Air-conducted click ABR
Air conduction (lower frequencies)	500-Hz toneburst ABR
Bone conduction	Bone-conducted click ABR

6.7. TEST PROTOCOLS FOR INFANTS AND CHILDREN

Our test protocol for all patients is a three-part method. We obtain responses to (a) clicks to assess the higher-frequency range, primarily 2000 to 4000 Hz; (b) 500-Hz tonebursts to assess the lower frequency range; and (c) bone-conducted clicks to distinguish between conductive and sensorineural hearing losses. Table 6–3 summarizes the test stimuli and what they evaluate.

When testing infants and children, ABRs are obtained for each of these stimuli. The test stimuli and test types are shown in Table 6–4.

We encourage use of two-channel four-electrode recordings, with electrodes placed at the vertex and at the medial side of each earlobe and a ground at the forehead. In infants, recording electrodes may be placed at the high forehead instead of the vertex and at the ipsilateral mastoid and/or C_7, as described in Chapter 7 on special considerations when testing infants.

6.7.1. ABR to Air-Conducted Clicks

Responses to air-conducted clicks are recorded for each ear individually. There are several methods that can be used to obtain the necessary information. We generally first obtain a response from each ear using 75-dB nHL 100-microsecond clicks in order to determine the latencies of Waves I, III, and V to assess neural integrity. In patients older than 18 months, adult normative values can be used in interpretation. In infants, we expect increased absolute and interwave latencies and use the normative data provided by Zimmerman et al. (1987). If no response is obtained at 75 dB nHL, then the click level is increased to the limits of the equipment to attempt to obtain a response.

We also obtain responses using both condensation and rarefaction clicks at a high intensity to compare responses obtained with each polarity. This is helpful in distinguishing the cochlear microphonic (which will reverse in phase as the stimulus does) from Wave I of the ABR (which will not show a phase reversal with clicks). Recently, we have observed a series of patients in our practice who, at high intensities, seem to show repeatable waves that turn out not to be an ABR, but a cochlear response (Berlin, 1996; Berlin et al., 1998). Thus, in patients where the entire response inverts when the polarity of the clicks is inverted, the "waves" represent a cochlear, not brainstem, response, and a neural disorder should be suspected (see Figure 4–2 and Case Study 17).

Following acquisition of responses at 75 dB nHL, the intensity of the click is decreased in 20-dB steps until no response is obtained. If the patient is quiet and we predict that sufficient time will be available to complete all parts of the test battery, then the click level may be increased by 10 dB to determine presence of a response at an intermediary level. For example, if responses are obtained at 75, 55, and 35 dB nHL, but no response is observed at 15 dB nHL, then stimuli are presented at 25 dB nHL. At higher intensities where responses are readily seen over the noise, fewer than 1000 averages may be sufficient. Closer to threshold, more than 2000 averages may be necessary.

Each of these responses is obtained twice to judge replicability and assist in determination of threshold. If the F_{SP} analysis method is available, then a second average for replication purposes may not be necessary. Latency of the response increases and amplitude decreases, quite predictably, with decreases in stimulus intensity. We generally are able to obtain responses to click stimuli at 15 to 25 dB nHL in infants and young children who have normal hearing and are quiet. An example of an intensity series for an air-conducted click obtained from an infant is shown in Figure 6–5. The Wave V latencies at each intensity are plotted onto an infant latency-intensity function in Figure 6–6. The infant latency-intensity function is further discussed in Chapter 7.

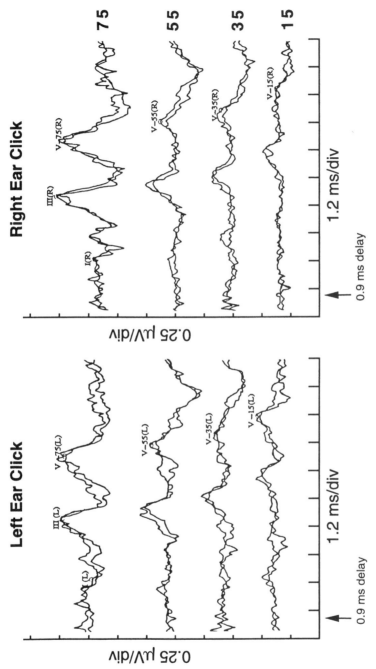

Figure 6-5. Intensity series for air-conducted click ABRs obtained in an infant.

107

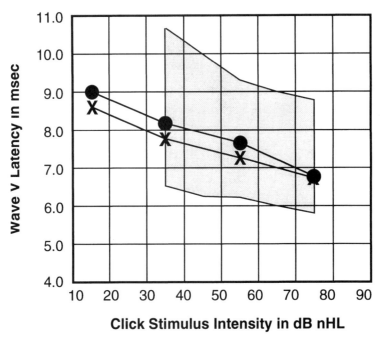

LATENCY-INTENSITY FUNCTION FOR INFANTS

Figure 6-6. Wave V absolute latencies from Figure 6-5 plotted as a function of intensity from 15 to 75 dB nHL. Note that absolute latencies are longer than those obtained in adults.

6.7.2. ABR to 500 Hz Tonebursts

ABRs obtained with click stimuli primarily provide information about hearing sensitivity in the 2000 to 4000 Hz range (e.g., Bauch & Olsen, 1986, 1987; Jerger, Hayes, & Jordan, 1980). Patients who have responses to clicks at normal levels may still have a low-frequency hearing loss. Patients who have elevated responses or no responses to clicks may have anything from normal hearing to a severe hearing loss in the low frequencies. Thus, click information is not sufficient to understand auditory function across the frequency range or to appropriately fit amplification. An ABR to a click alone cannot differentiate among the audiograms showing either low-frequency or high-frequency hearing loss (Figure 6–7). For the audiograms in the left panel of Figure 6–7, click responses would be normal or near normal, despite the varying degrees of low-frequency hearing loss. The right panel shows higher frequency hearing loss configurations associated with various click thresholds. Without low-frequency toneburst data, the overall hearing configuration could be falling (as shown here), flat, or rising. Acquisition of responses to low-frequency stimuli is necessary to define the configuration of hearing sensitivity. We have found the ABR with a 500-Hz toneburst

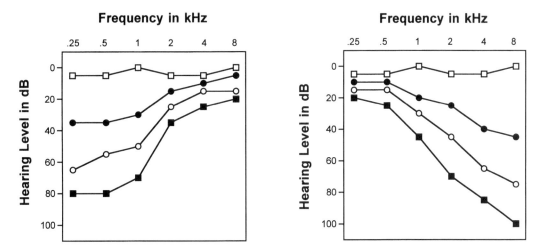

Figure 6–7. Audiograms showing four different configurations of low-frequency hearing loss (left panel) and four different degrees of high-frequency hearing loss (right panel).

Table 6–5. Test parameters for 500-Hz toneburst ABR.

Test Parameter	Setting
Stimulus	
Center frequency	500 Hz
Duration (cycles)	2-0-2 cycles (rise-plateau-fall)
Duration (ms)	4-0-4 ms (rise-plateau-fall)
Stimulus polarity	Condensation
Stimulus rate	39.1/s
Time window	
Infants	25 ms
Adults	20 ms
Filter bandwidth	30–1500 Hz
Number of sweeps[a]	1000–2000
Number of replications	At least 2

[a]Generally, fewer sweeps are necessary at higher intensities whereas more sweeps are necessary at lower intensities.

stimulus very effective, though other low-frequency stimuli, such as 250 Hz tonebursts, may also be used.

For 500-Hz toneburst ABRs, we set the filter cutoffs from 30 to 1500 Hz in order to accommodate lower frequency physiological activity (see Table 6–5). Tonebursts with 4-ms (two cycles) rise and fall times, Hanning or Blackmann stimulus envelopes, and either condensation or rarefaction polarity (but not alternating polarity) are used.

The time window is extended to 20 or 25 ms because these responses have longer latencies than responses to clicks. Stimuli are presented at a rate near but not at 40 per second (e.g., 39.1 per second) to each ear individually beginning at 75 dB nHL and then decreasing in 20- (or sometimes 10-) dB steps until no response is obtained.

Among the many important considerations in presenting toneburst stimuli is the use of a single-polarity stimulus. As discussed in Section 6.5.2, peak latencies shift when the polarity of the stimulus is reversed, particularly for lower frequency stimuli (see Figure 6–3). Use of alternating-polarity stimuli with lower frequency stimuli can result in amplitude reduction and sometimes complete obliteration of the toneburst ABR. Because ABR toneburst testing most often involves low-frequency stimuli, use of either rarefaction or condensation tonebursts is especially important. Condensation polarity stimuli often result in higher amplitude later ABR components than rarefaction stimuli. Therefore, we recommend use of condensation tonebursts because it is the later components that remain at intensities near threshold.

When interpreting the responses obtained to 500-Hz tonebursts, we look for a single replicable peak that represents Wave V of the ABR. We generally observe a single peak that may have a sinusoidal overlay at high intensities. An example of an ABR intensity series from an adult obtained with 500-Hz tonebursts is shown in Figure 6–8. The typical five- to seven-wave complex seen with clicks (e.g., ABRs with Waves I, III, and V) generally is not seen in responses obtained with these low-frequency stimuli.

Peak latencies range from 6 to 10 ms for high-intensity stimuli to 10 to 16 ms nearer threshold (Gorga, Kaminski, Beauchaine, & Jesteadt, 1988). Figure 6–9 shows mean response latency (and one standard deviation) as a function of intensity from 10 of our normative adult subjects for 500-Hz tonebursts with 4-2-4 ms and 2-1-2 ms envelopes. Note that the latencies for the 2-1-2 ms stimuli are shorter, which is consistent with the more rapid rise time. In infants, these latencies will be even longer. In our experience, thresholds of ABRs to 500-Hz tonebursts obtained from normal-hearing individuals using the test parameters shown here are generally between 25 and 35 dB nHL (above behavioral threshold; e.g., Hood & Berlin, 1986). Responses in normal ears are only sometimes seen for stimuli below 25 dB nHL.

6.7.3. ABR to Bone-Conducted Clicks

When responses to air-conducted clicks and tonebursts are present at normal threshold levels, there is no need to obtain bone-conducted responses, as in

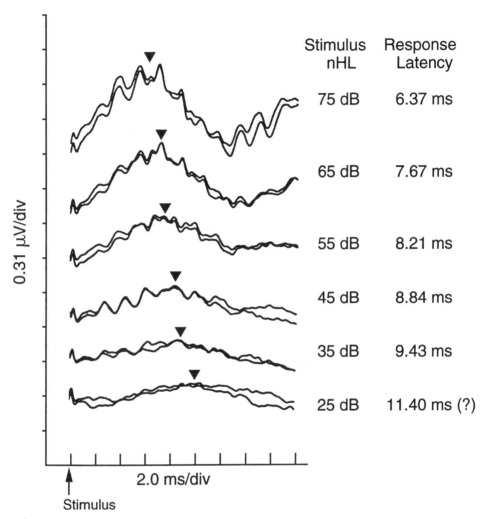

Stimulus nHL	Response Latency
75 dB	6.37 ms
65 dB	7.67 ms
55 dB	8.21 ms
45 dB	8.84 ms
35 dB	9.43 ms
25 dB	11.40 ms (?)

0.31 µV/div

2.0 ms/div

Stimulus

Figure 6-8. ABR intensity series obtained with 500-Hz tonebursts in a normal individual. Stimuli ranged from 25 to 75 dB nHL; response latencies are marked with inverted triangles.

conventional audiometry. However, when either the click or 500-Hz toneburst responses are not present at expected normal levels, then ABRs should be completed using bone-conducted clicks. Clicks are presented at progressively decreasing intensities via bone conduction to determine whether there is a difference in levels at which responses are obtained between air and bone conduction. If such a discrepancy does exist, this suggests the presence of a conductive or mixed hearing loss.

The test parameters for bone-conducted clicks used are the same as those for air-conducted clicks except that this is the one instance where we use alternating-

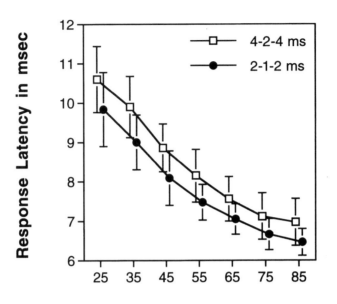

Toneburst Intensity in dB nHL

Figure 6–9. Response latencies for 500-Hz tonebursts as a function of stimulus intensity. Data are shown for tonebursts with 4-ms rise, 2-ms plateau, and 4-ms fall times and for stimuli with 2-ms rise, 1-ms plateau, and 2-ms fall times. Latencies are shorter for the briefer stimuli. Bars represent ± one standard deviation.

polarity stimuli (Table 6–6). The reason for use of alternating-polarity clicks in bone conduction testing is the large electrical artifact emitted from the bone oscillator. Oscillator placement can be at either the forehead or mastoid. We use mastoid placement in infants because stimuli from the bone oscillator are conducted across the scalp less efficiently in infants than in adults (Yang, Stuart, Mencher, Mencher, & Vincer, 1993).

The spectrum of the bone-conducted click is somewhat different than that of air-conducted clicks due to differences in the frequency responses of the two transducers. More importantly, the dynamic range is different, as is true in audiometric application. The dynamic range of the bone-conducted stimuli rarely exceeds 45 to 55 dB, and the relationship between the output of the oscillator and the "dial reading" varies with different instruments. Thus, it is important to determine what the dial reading means and how this relates to the oscillator output.

Stimuli are presented beginning at the highest output level (usually about 50 dB nHL) and then decreased in 20-dB steps as in the other tests. Responses are first obtained without masking and then, if response thresholds are better than those obtained by air conduction and/or there is asymmetry between ears, masking with broadband noise is used.

Table 6-6. Test parameters for air-conducted and bone-conducted clicks when used to estimate hearing sensitivity.

Test Parameter	Air-Conducted Clicks	Bone-Conducted Clicks
Stimulus	100-μs pulse	100-μs pulse
Stimulus polarity		
High intensity	Condensation *and* rarefaction	Alternating
Lower intensities	Condensation *or* rarefaction	Alternating
Stimulus rate		
Initial	27.7/s	27.7/s
Slow (if 27.7/s response poor)	7.7/s	
Time window		
Infants	15 ms	15 ms
Adults	10 or 12 ms	10 or 12 ms
Filter bandwidth		
Standard	100–3000 Hz	100–3000 Hz
Emphasis of Wave V	30–3000 Hz	30–3000 Hz
Number of sweeps[a]	1000–2000	1000–2000
Number of replications[b]	At least 2	At least 2

[a]Generally, fewer sweeps are necessary at higher intensities whereas more sweeps are necessary at lower intensities. Use of F_{SP} estimates is recommended when available.
[b]Replications are not necessary when F_{SP} method is used.

Because the output in bone conduction is limited, the responses obtained by bone conduction will rarely show the familiar five-wave complex seen at high intensities in standard air-conduction ABRs. Responses will resemble those obtained with air-conducted clicks in the response threshold to 50-dB nHL range. Because we are interested only in determining the presence and threshold of the response, Wave V is the only component necessary to assess. An example of an intensity series obtained for bone-conducted clicks is shown in Figure 6–10.

6.8. MODIFICATIONS TO IMPROVE TEST EFFICIENCY

Several modifications can be used to improve test efficiency by decreasing test time. Some instruments have the capability to estimate signal-to-noise levels with either an F_{SP} statistic or another method of signal-to-noise ratio estimation. These methods may require fewer averages, reduce the need to replicate the response, and provide an objective estimate of response presence (e.g., Sininger, 1993). Another method uses very high stimulus rates (on the order of 500–1000 stimuli per second) with randomized presentation sequences, known as maximum length sequences (e.g., Picton et al., 1992). Different sequences can be

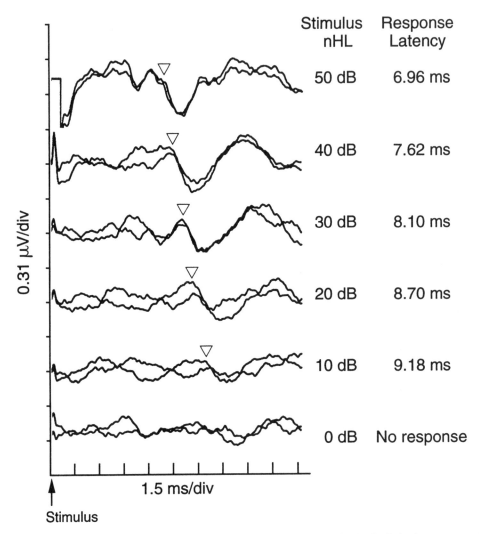

Figure 6-10. ABR intensity series obtained with bone-conducted clicks in a normal individual. Wave V latencies are marked for stimuli from 10 to 50 dB nHL.

presented to each ear, which allows testing of both ears simultaneously; when coupled with fast presentation rates, this greatly decreases overall test time. We find both of these techniques useful in our practice. Further descriptions are provided in Section 3.4 in Chapter 3.

Two other methods that can be used with any evoked potential system are a binaural-monaural combination of presentation and use of rapid, but not overlapping, stimulus rates. Jerger, Oliver, and Stach (1985) recommended using binaural stimuli at high and low intensities to quickly focus on response threshold. Stimuli are first presented in the 75–80 dB nHL range and then the stimulus intensity is immediately decreased to about 25 dB nHL for the second set of averages. If responses are present at both intensities, then one knows that at least one ear has a normal synchrony and sensitivity. Then, each ear can be tested individually by presenting stimuli at about 10 dB above the lowest level where the binaural response was obtained. The purpose of this procedure is to reduce the number of "runs" necessary to locate the threshold of the response.

Picton (1978) recommended the use of faster stimulus rates when in the threshold-seeking mode of testing. Presenting stimuli on the order of 50–70 clicks per second will reduce test time. Although Wave V latency is prolonged, the amplitude is not reduced as much as earlier components, making acquisition of responses near threshold possible.

6.9. TEST PROTOCOL FOR OLDER CHILDREN AND ADULTS USING THE 40-Hz RESPONSE

The test protocol used for older children (over 8 to 10 years of age) who are not sedated and for adults varies only slightly from that used for infants and children. The reason for the modification is test efficiency. The same stimuli (clicks and 500-Hz tonebursts) are used and ABRs are obtained in the same manner for air- and bone-conducted clicks. The recording technique for the 500-Hz toneburst is the 40-Hz response, which is more similar to a middle latency response.

First described by Galambos, Makeig, and Talmachoff (1981), this response has not been found useful in infants and young children due to effects of maturation and sedation. However, the 40-Hz response is quite useful in older children and adults for estimating auditory sensitivity using low-frequency stimuli (Stapells, Linden, Suffield, Hamel, & Picton, 1984). The test parameters used in older children and adults are summarized in Table 6–7.

The 40-Hz response denotes the type of response obtained and should not be confused with the stimulus used, which is the same toneburst as used when

Table 6–7. Three-part test protocol for the estimation of hearing sensitivity in older children and adults.

Stimulus/Target	Response
Air conduction (higher frequencies)	Air-conducted click ABR
Air conduction (lower frequencies)	40-Hz response using a 500-Hz toneburst stimulus
Bone conduction	Bone-conducted click ABR

Table 6-8. Test parameters for 40-Hz response with 500-Hz toneburst.

Test Parameter	Setting
Stimulus	
Center frequency	500 Hz
Duration (cycles)	2-0-2 cycles (rise-plateau-fall)
Duration (ms)	4-0-4 ms (rise-plateau-fall)
Stimulus polarity	Condensation
Stimulus rate	39.1/s
Time window	100 ms
Filter bandwidth	5–100 Hz or 10–100 Hz
Number of sweeps[a]	200–400
Number of replications	At least 2

[a]Generally, fewer sweeps are necessary at higher intensities whereas more sweeps are necessary at lower intensities.

acquiring the 500-Hz toneburst ABR. This evoked potential uses a relatively fast presentation rate (about 40 stimuli per second) and, because of its higher amplitude, usually requires only about 200 sweeps, making it possible to obtain responses in a few seconds. Test speed and the ability to obtain responses near behavioral threshold make it a desirable technique for estimating auditory sensitivity.

The 40-Hz response is best obtained using a presentation rate near (e.g., 39.1 or 40.3 stimuli per second), but not at, 40 stimuli per second. The response, recorded across a 100-ms time period, resembles a sinusoidal wave with peaks occurring about every 25 ms. The spectral translation (fast Fourier transform) of the waveform is approximately 40 Hz, which provides the basis for the name of the evoked potential as the 40-Hz response. As noted in Table 6–8, some of the test parameters (filters, time window) are similar to those used in acquiring middle-latency responses. Other characteristics of the 40-Hz response are similar to the middle-latency response as well. For example, this response is not mature in young patients and thus not applicable in infants and young children. It is adversely affected by sedation or sleep and thus is best recorded in awake patients.

The 40-Hz response is characterized by four broad peaks across a 100-ms time window (Figure 6–11). The amplitude of the response decreases as stimulus intensity decreases, but there is little change in peak latency (Figure 6–12). In distinguishing the presence or absence of a response, we look for replicable responses with at least three of four peaks present at intervals of approximately 25 ms. The threshold of the 40-Hz response coincides with behavioral thresholds within about 10 dB (Galambos et al., 1981). In the example shown in Figure 6–12,

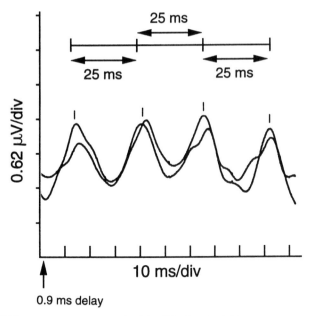

Figure 6-11. 40-Hz responses recorded to 75-dB nHL 500-Hz tonebursts. Positive and negative peaks in the response occur approximately every 25 ms.

a response was present at 5 dB nHL. Although we use 500-Hz stimuli when acquiring the 40-Hz response, other frequency tonebursts can be used as well.

6.10. STEADY-STATE RESPONSES

Recently, additional types of evoked potentials, obtained using frequency-modulated and amplitude-modulated tones, have been studied (Picton, Skinner, Champagne, Kellet, & Maiste, 1987; Rickards & Clark, 1984). These responses are generally referred to as steady state responses (SSRs) or steady state evoked potentials (SSEPs).

Unlike ABRs obtained with click stimuli, SSRs or SSEPs use stimuli that are continuous tones. Modulation of the tones over time in either the frequency or amplitude domain results in small frequency or amplitude changes in the stimuli. It is the responses of the neural system to these changes, or modulations, in the stimuli that can be recorded. The stimuli are modulated tones, so the stimulus has very good frequency specificity because spectral energy is contained only at the frequency of the carrier tone and the frequency of the modulation.

Responses to these stimuli are recorded at stimulus rates between 75 and 110 stimuli per second (or 75 to 110 Hz). As with the 40-Hz response, a fast stimulus

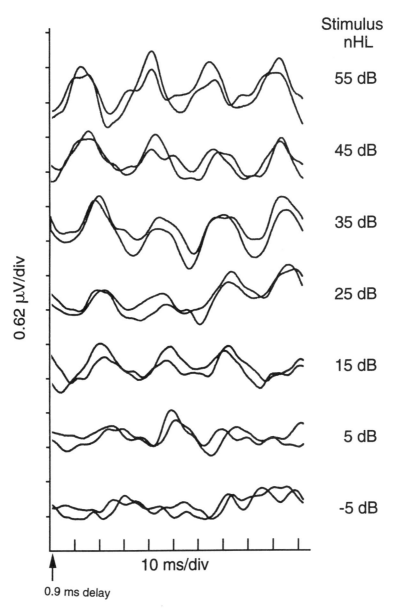

Figure 6-12. 40-Hz responses recorded to 500-Hz tonebursts at intensity levels of -5 to 55 dB nHL. Responses are present at 5 dB nHL and above.

rate is used in which the responses to stimuli overlap. Unlike the 40-Hz response, these steady-state responses are unaffected by sleep and can be recorded in young children and infants (Cohen, Rickards, & Clark, 1991; Lins & Picton, 1995).

The use of relatively rapid stimulus rates improves test efficiency over standard recording techniques. In addition, different frequency stimuli (e.g., 500, 1000, 2000, and 4000 Hz) can be presented simultaneously, with each frequency modulated at a slightly different rate. Little change in amplitude over presentation of single frequencies is observed (Lins & Picton, 1995). With proper instrumentation, it is also possible to test both ears simultaneously by applying different modulation rates to stimuli routed to each ear. In clinical practice, stimuli can be presented at various intensities in order to estimate the lowest intensity where a response is evident.

There are several characteristics of the SSEP, or SSR, that make it potentially a very useful clinical technique. The amplitude and phase of the response at the frequency of modulation can be measured automatically by a computer. A composite of responses to stimuli at various frequencies and intensities can be constructed in order to view the lowest levels where responses are obtained, much as in the construction of an audiogram. Thus identification of peaks is not necessary and objective procedures for response identification can be used.

Comparisons of response thresholds to behavioral thresholds show that responses can be obtained at about 10 to 20 dB above behavioral thresholds using carrier tones between 500 and 4000 Hz. Generally, better agreement is obtained for higher than lower frequency tones and closer agreement is observed in persons with hearing loss than those with normal hearing (Lins et al., 1996; Rance, Rickards, Cohen, De Vidi, & Clark, 1995).

A further potential benefit of steady-state responses is its potential application in the evaluation of hearing aids. Amplitude-modulated tones are not significantly distorted by sound-field speakers and are of sufficient duration to allow appropriate processing through hearing aids (T. W. Picton, personal communication, 1998).

6.11. SN$_{10}$ RESPONSE

H. Davis and Hirsh (1979) described a vertex-negative potential (SN$_{10}$) that occurs at a latency of approximately 10 ms for a 60-dB nHL stimulus. Latency for a 500-Hz toneburst at approximately 15 dB above threshold is near 15 ms. Although the SN$_{10}$ response is not widely used clinically at present, it provides an interesting historical perspective to the evolution of use of the brainstem response in estimating hearing sensitivity.

To record the SN$_{10}$ response, Davis recommended use of a 2-1-2 period envelope, a low-frequency filter cutoff of 30 or 50 Hz, and a high-frequency cutoff of 3000 Hz with a 24-dB-per-octave slope. The SN$_{10}$ response is best observed with a filter of 24 dB per octave, and, according to the report of Stapells and Picton (1981), who compared various filter slopes, there is a reversal in the most recognizable component at low intensities when filter slopes are changed from 12 dB per octave to 24 dB per octave.

H. Davis et al. (1985) reported that the P6 (Wave V)-SN_{10} combination was most efficient in identifying responses at 500, 1000, 2000, and 4000 Hz. Evoked potential thresholds were generally obtained within 10 dB of behavioral thresholds, although ranges of from 0 to 35 dB have been reported for the slow wave response (Klein, 1983). Hawes and Greenberg (1981) reported that the SN_{10} was identifiable in newborns as well as in adults. Responses from subjects in their study occurred more often for clicks and for 1000-Hz and 2000-Hz tonebursts than for 500-Hz tonebursts.

6.12. USE OF MASKING

When using clicks and tonebursts to assess hearing sensitivity, masking should be used when sensitivity differences between ears are suspected or observed. Broadband noise should be used when the stimuli are clicks. As in pure-tone audiometry, narrowband masking may provide more effective masking of tonebursts than broadband masking. If a narrowband masking stimulus is not available on the evoked potential system, then narrowband noise provided through an audiometer can be used as long as effective masking levels for the toneburst stimuli are established.

6.13. RELATION OF RESPONSES TO BEHAVIORAL THRESHOLDS

Evoked potentials obtained using clicks and tonebursts have been compared to pure-tone behavioral thresholds. Several investigators have compared various frequency combinations and reported that clicks were most consistent with thresholds in the 2000 to 4000 Hz range (Bauch & Olsen, 1986, 1987; Jerger, Hayes, & Jordan, 1980). The threshold of the click-elicited ABR agrees with behavioral thresholds within a range of 6 to 20 dB (e.g., Coats & Martin, 1977; Jerger & Mauldin, 1978; K. Møller & Blegvad, 1976; Newton & Barratt, 1983; Pratt & Sohmer, 1978; Smith & Simmons, 1982).

Responses to 500-Hz tonebursts can be observed at intensities within approximately 10 to 25 dB of behavioral threshold. Wave V is the component of the ABR that is considered most recognizable at low intensities (Bauch, Rose, & Harner, 1980). Longer latencies should be expected for lower frequency stimuli (e.g., Bauch et al., 1980; Beattie, Moretti, & Warren, 1984; Fowler & Noffsinger, 1983; Kodera, Yamane, Yamada, & Suzuki, 1977). The latency differences between low- and high-frequency tonebursts and among various studies are highly dependent on the differences in stimulus duration and thus spectral content.

Table 6–9. Considerations when using the ABR to estimate hearing sensitivity.

Factor	Description
Neural integrity	An intact neural system is necessary
Collapsing ear canals	Check for or use insert earphones
Middle ear status	Tympanograms and MEMRs are helpful in interpretation and as a cross-check
Otoacoustic emissions	Helpful in distinguishing peripheral sensory from neural disorder when no ABR is present
The ABR is not a hearing test	Although not a direct test of hearing, the ABR is very useful in estimating peripheral hearing sensitivity

Note: MEMR = middle ear muscle reflex.

6.14. CAUTIONS AND CONSIDERATIONS

As with any physiological or behavioral test, there are a number of factors to keep in mind in order to make appropriate application of the test and correctly interpret test results. Some the many factors that we consider when using auditory evoked potentials are listed in Table 6–9.

6.14.1. Neural Integrity

Measuring auditory evoked potentials requires an *intact neural system.* Thus, abnormalities that can affect the neural system must be considered in interpretation of test results. For example, in the presence of hydrocephalus, the ABR can be obliterated despite normal hearing. Infants and adults with an auditory neuropathy (distinguished by an absent ABR even though otoacoustic emissions are present) underscore the *importance of obtaining otoacoustic emissions in patients who fail to show an ABR at any intensity.* Presence of an ABR at high intensities but not to lower intensity stimuli is consistent with a peripheral hearing loss. Absence of an ABR to high and low intensities may mean either a peripheral hearing loss or a neural disorder. Otoacoustic emissions can be helpful in *separating peripheral hearing loss from some neural disorders.*

6.14.2. Collapsing Ear Canals

We always use insert earphones to avoid the possibility of collapsing ear canals. Insert earphones are more comfortable, which may enhance a patient's state of relaxation or sleep.

6.14.3. Middle Ear Function and Otoacoustic Emissions

Part of our test battery always includes tympanograms and middle ear muscle reflexes as well as otoacoustic emissions. If the patient requires sedation (as in the case of most infants over about 4 months of age and young children), then it is important to obtain these measures *before* doing the ABR. During sedated deep sleep, *positive pressure may build up in the middle ears,* which can compromise the results of middle-ear measures and otoacoustic emissions.

6.14.4. The ABR Is Not a Hearing Test

Finally, it is always important to remember that the ABR *is not a direct test of hearing.* In those patients who do not have good neural synchrony, other means of estimating auditory function must be sought. In addition, *passing an ABR as an infant does not preclude the possibility of acquired or later onset hereditary hearing loss.* Thus, in reporting test results, we always inform parents and referral sources of the importance of monitoring children's speech and language development and observing their responses to their auditory environment. Should a child fail to develop speech and language, parents are advised to seek appropriate evaluation and management. In those individuals with ABR results consistent with peripheral hearing loss, management is initiated based on ABR and other test results, with the ultimate goal of obtaining behavioral hearing test information when possible.

6.15. TECHNICAL ERRORS

Some of the limitations of the ABR are related to technical problems that result from improper test setup or procedures. A checklist of technical considerations is shown in Table 6–10.

Table 6-10. Checklist for appropriate test techniques.

Stimulus:	_____ Type (click, toneburst)
	_____ Intensity
	_____ Duration
	_____ Envelope
	_____ Calibration
	_____ Transducer (earphone, bone oscillator)
	_____ Ear canal collapse
Response:	_____ Amplification
	_____ Filter band
	_____ Time window
	_____ Artifact rejection
Subject:	_____ Electrode preparation and placement
	_____ Electrode impedance low and balanced
	_____ Electrodes correctly connected
	_____ Instructions
	_____ Quiet and relaxed

Careful control of stimulus intensity and stimulus delivery is necessary to ensure appropriate data for analysis of waveform latencies and of response thresholds. Ear canal collapse (Ventry et al., 1962) or earphone slippage can reduce signal intensity at the ear without the examiner's knowledge. Improperly calibrated stimuli can also compromise test accuracy.

Technical errors in equipment setup, such as inappropriate electrode routing or inappropriate amplification of the biological signal, may result in erroneous recordings. The filter band and time window should be appropriate for the response the clinician wishes to record. The artifact rejection system may be set at a rejection level so sensitive that the signal one wishes to record exceeds the artifact rejection limits.

Improper subject preparation can result in noisy or difficult to interpret recordings. Poor electrode impedance or dissimilar impedances among electrodes may yield poorly defined, difficult to interpret responses. Subjects who are very tense, not advised of the need to relax, or placed in an uncomfortable position or environment may produce excessive muscle artifact.

7

Testing Infants and Children With Physiological Measures

7.1. PHYSIOLOGICAL TECHNIQUES IN PEDIATRIC AUDIOLOGY

Physiological measures take on particular importance when evaluating the integrity of the auditory system in infants and children. Although physiological techniques cannot measure the "moment of hearing," they have proved useful in determining the mechanical and neural integrity of the auditory system, which are critical factors for normal hearing.

This chapter presents a broader view of the use of the auditory brainstem response (ABR) along with other physiological methods of assessing auditory function. Use of the ABR to estimate hearing sensitivity is an *indirect* approach to ascertaining true auditory function. Thus, a test battery approach is of paramount importance. In infants and young children, in whom physiological test results cannot be immediately corroborated by behavioral information, clinicians can use combinations of physiological measures to obtain as much information as possible and use each of these measures as cross-checks of the information each test provides to obtain a cohesive view of auditory function.

Several objective, physiological techniques are available to the clinician to determine the functional integrity of the auditory system from the middle ear to the cortex. The most commonly used measures include middle ear immittance and middle ear muscle reflexes (MEMRs), otoacoustic emissions, and auditory evoked potentials. Newborn infants and some toddlers and children cannot provide reliable behavioral responses to auditory stimuli. Even when reliable behavioral responses are obtained, physiological measures can provide additional important information. Thus, using physiological measures either as the primary measure or as a cross-check with other tests is valuable in these populations.

7.2. IMMITTANCE AND MIDDLE EAR MUSCLE REFLEXES

Middle ear measurements of immittance and the MEMR provide important information about the integrity of the middle ear system and the neural reflex arc through the lower brainstem pathways that carry information to elicit contraction of the stapedius muscle. These measures are considered an integral part of the basic hearing evaluation in audiological practice and are particularly important in infants and children due to the higher incidence of middle ear disorders in these groups.

Middle ear tests are effective in testing for middle ear pathology, determining the presence or absence of MEMRs, and evaluating facial nerve function. To make appropriate interpretation of the results, it is essential to keep in mind exactly what is being measured and to understand both the advantages and limits of each component of the middle ear test battery. Immittance measures the mechanical properties of the auditory path from the external ear to the stapedial footplate. Because flexible external ear tissues and partly formed or immature canal walls can give spurious results, care must be taken when completing these measures in infants. This, however, does not mean that these measures should not be used. If normal tympanograms (particularly if multifrequency tympanometry is completed) and MEMRs are obtained, then it is highly likely that there are no middle ear pathologies and that the infant does not have a severe hearing loss. In contrast, a normal-appearing tympanogram with absent MEMRs may suggest a severe or profound hearing loss but may also be misleading due to flexible ear canal geometry that could simulate a normal tympanogram when using a 220-Hz tone.

Middle ear tests are best used in conjunction with the ABR and/or a full audiological test battery. They provide a useful cross-check for other clinical measures of the middle ear, cochlea, and lower brainstem pathways. When using middle ear measures in sedated infants or children, immittance and MEMRs should be completed *before* beginning the ABR because positive pressure in the middle ear may build up over time in infants or children who snore or breathe heavily during sedated sleep. If middle ear pressure does deviate from normal over the period of time needed to complete the ABR, then the validity of the middle ear measures will be compromised. Experience has shown that MEMRs can be measured in most sedated infants and children without awakening them.

When no MEMR responses are obtained, testing for presence of nonacoustic reflexes should be completed. It is erroneous to think that absence of a stapedius reflex response due to physical absence of the middle ear muscles themselves is common. Nonacoustic reflexes can be elicited by a puff of air to the eye or a gentle rub of a wisp of cotton in the anterior tragal region. If there is contraction of the middle ear muscles to nonacoustic stimulation but no contraction to acoustic stimulation, this is not a normal variation and should be considered a pathologic sign.

Patterns among middle ear measurements and other test results can provide important insights into auditory function. For example, it is highly unlikely that a patient who has no response behaviorally to sound is physiologically deaf if MEMRs are present at levels between 70 and 80 dB HL. Conversely, a child who appears to give behavioral responses in the normal-hearing or mild hearing loss ranges and has normal tympanograms but no MEMRs is still highly suspect for a severe hearing loss. The exceptions to this possibility are in young infants, as noted above, and in patients with an auditory neuropathy. Also, normal MEMRs often are obtained in patients with mild or moderate cochlear losses, so normal reflex responses cannot rule out hearing losses in this range.

7.3. EVOKED OTOACOUSTIC EMISSIONS

Evoked otoacoustic emissions (EOAEs) have several clinical applications when evaluating newborns, infants, and children. Types of EOAEs that are used extensively clinically are click-evoked otoacoustic emissions and distortion product emissions. EOAEs are widely used in screening programs to rule out hearing loss in newborn infants, and EOAEs and ABR are considered standards for this purpose by many audiologists and many other health care professionals. EOAEs are growing in importance as part of the clinical test battery and as a cross-check to behavioral tests, middle ear measures, and evoked potential results.

Otoacoustic emissions are particularly robust in infants who are free of external and/ or middle ear pathology (Kemp, Ryan, & Bray, 1990; Lafreniere, Smurzynski, Jung, Leonard, & Kim, 1993). This characteristic makes EOAEs particularly useful in this population; and even though infants are often physiologically "noisier" than adults, the higher amplitude of the EOAEs allows their acquisition while maintaining acceptable signal-to-noise relationships (see Figure 7–1). EOAE amplitude increases from newborn to ages of from 1 to 9 months, whereas decreases in amplitude have been observed in children aged 4–13 years, with an average amplitude for click EOAEs of 15 dB SPL in that age range (Norton & Widen, 1990; Widen, 1997).

Otoacoustic emissions are expected to be present in ears that have hearing sensitivity that is better than approximately 30 to 40 dB HL, with an absence of any external or middle ear pathologies. Thus, EOAEs can be used as a screening measure to determine whether a hearing loss may be present. Because physical characteristics of the external and middle ears can influence the amplitude of emissions, actual hearing sensitivity cannot be readily predicted. Emissions have been shown to fluctuate with cochlear hearing loss and to provide information about the configuration of hearing loss, and they are used in monitoring the effects of ototoxic medications. Otoacoustic emissions also have particular value, when used in conjunction with the ABR, in identifying patients with an auditory neuropathy. The ease of recording emissions, their generally robust nature, and their reliability contribute to their value as a clinical test.

7.4. AUDITORY EVOKED POTENTIALS

7.4.1. Auditory Brainstem Response

7.4.1.1. Who Should Be Tested?

ABR testing is indicated in infants who are at risk for hearing loss or neurological problems or who have congenital atresia or other aural deformities (Finitzo-Hieber, Hecox, & Cone, 1979); older children with developmental delays and/or multiple handicaps (e.g., Stein et al., 1987); deaf-blind patients (Stein, Özdamar,

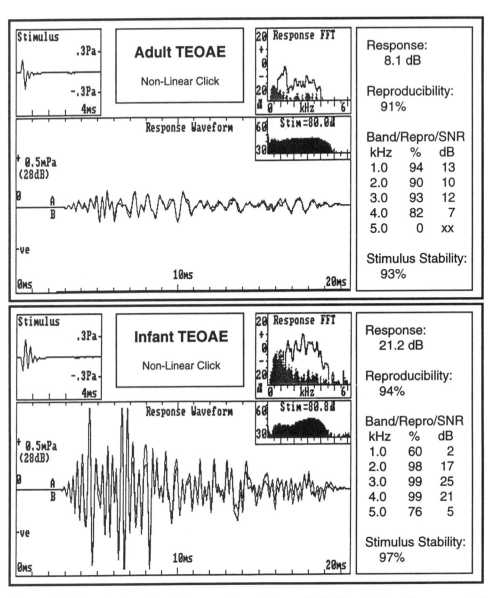

Figure 7-1. Transient-evoked otoacoustic emissions (TEOAEs) obtained from an adult (*top panel*) and an infant (*bottom panel*) using 80-dB peak sound pressure nonlinear clicks. Note higher amplitude in the infant TEOAE.

& Schnabel, 1981); patients with delayed language; difficult to test children; and patients with suspected degenerative disorders (Jacobson & Hecox, 1982; Mokotoff, Schulman-Galambos, & Galambos, 1977; Schulman-Galambos & Galambos, 1979; Starr et al., 1977). ABR testing has been used as a prognostic indicator in cases of asphyxia, perinatal hypoxia/ischemia, hyperbilirubinemia, congenital cranial and facial anomalies, and intracranial hemorrhage (Hecox &

Cone, 1981; Stockard & Stockard, 1981). Student and Sohmer (1978) suggested that ABRs in autistic patients are characterized by prolonged Wave I latency and prolonged interwave latencies.

7.4.1.2. Estimating Auditory Sensitivity in Infants and Children

A comprehensive ABR test protocol is described in Chapter 6. This protocol includes responses to (a) air-conducted clicks to assess the higher frequency range, primarily 2000–4000 Hz; (b) low-frequency (generally 500 Hz) tonebursts to assess the lower frequency range; and (c) bone-conducted clicks to distinguish between conductive and sensorineural hearing losses. The test parameters and procedures used at Kresge Hearing Research Laboratory and its associated clinics are described in Chapter 6.

7.4.1.3. Examining Auditory Pathway Integrity

Auditory evoked potentials are useful in the evaluation of neural integrity in children who present with suspected auditory processing problems. Determining the presence or absence of functional abnormalities in the neural pathways can be done to support observed behavioral difficulties with auditory tasks. To accomplish this, a combination of ABR, middle latency responses, and cortical potentials can be used.

When ABR testing is completed, even though the overall purpose of the testing may be to obtain information about hearing sensitivity, replicable responses should be obtained at an intensity level that allows identification of Waves I, III, and V in order to evaluate absolute and interwave latencies and assess responses from a neural standpoint. Although immaturity of the neural pathways must be considered in patients below 12 to 18 months of age, the clinician should look for presence of response components and general relationships of responses obtained from each ear. A comparison of infant and adult ABRs with peak latencies marked is shown in Figure 7–2. ABRs in infants younger than 12 to 18 months are distinguished from those obtained from older children and adults by latency, amplitude, and morphological differences. Absolute latencies of the later ABR components are more prolonged than earlier waves in infants, resulting in longer interwave latencies. Amplitude differences also may exist in infants where Waves I and III are more prominent than Wave V.

7.4.2. Middle Latency and Late Potentials

The middle latency response (MLR) and cortical potentials have been used in objective determination of hearing thresholds, assessment of auditory pathway function and localization of lesions, and assessment of cochlear implant function. Middle latency responses and cortical potentials are affected by sleep and sedation, are susceptible to muscle activity, and have a longer neuromaturational time

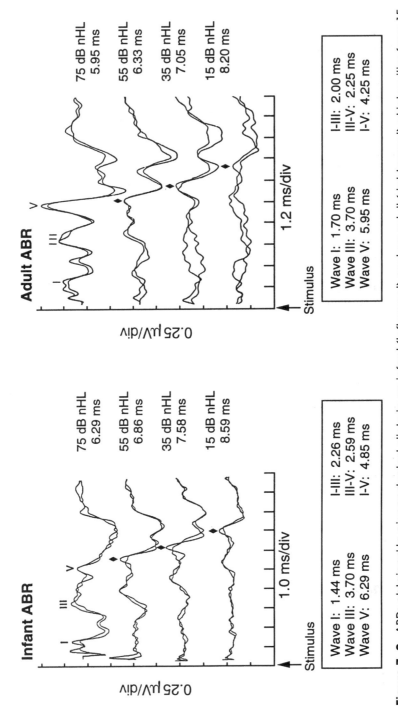

Figure 7-2. ABRs obtained to air-conducted clicks in an infant (left panel) and an adult (right panel) at intensities from 15 to 75 dB nHL. Note longer absolute and interwave latencies in the infant responses and differences in waveform morphology.

course than the ABR. Although these potentials may be more difficult to record reliably in young children, researchers and clinicians have developed various techniques to distract or involve children who are awake according to the requirements of the protocol. An excellent discussion of the characteristics and sources of the middle and late potentials can be found in Kraus and McGee (1992).

Responses that reflect ability to distinguish between stimuli appear promising in evaluating and understanding various aspects of auditory perception in children. Cortical potentials such as the P300 response and mismatch negativity (MMN) are *event-related potentials* that occur when the brain makes a decision about whether one stimulus differs from another. For these responses, two different stimuli are presented randomly with one of the stimuli occurring only rarely. The patient's task in recording the P300 response is to count the number of "different" or rarely occurring stimuli. Mismatch negativity responses use a similar stimulus paradigm, but are recorded without participation of the patient, other than remaining quiet, and thus may be more suited to pediatric populations. Mismatch negativity responses have been recorded reliably in school-age children and appear to be a promising technique in understanding various auditory perception abilities in children, assessing the effectiveness of cochlear implants, and monitoring the effectiveness of intervention programs (Kraus, McGee, Carrell, & Sharma, 1995).

7.4.3. Strengths and Limitations of Auditory Evoked Potentials in Pediatric Applications

Auditory evoked potentials, when used and interpreted properly, provide a powerful method of evaluating neural status and obtaining reliable estimates of auditory sensitivity in infants, young children, and other individuals who cannot participate in behavioral testing or provide reliable behavioral responses. Auditory evoked potentials also can provide an important physiological cross-check of behavioral test results. Table 7–1 summarizes strengths and limitations of the ABR in newborn and infant testing.

7.4.3.1. Strengths

A search for hearing loss and deafness in infants can be performed at or soon after birth. Immaturity of the nervous system must be taken into account, but the ability to study neurological status as well as hearing sensitivity allows a suitable intervention process to begin at an early age. The ABR is not affected by sleep or sedation, making it particularly useful in pediatric applications.

Frequency-specific testing is possible through use of several different stimulus and recording paradigms. While not as frequency specific as pure tones, information about the general audiometric configuration can be obtained. Some

Table 7-1. Strengths and limitations of the ABR in newborn and infant testing.

Strengths	Limitations
Can test at or soon after birth	Need to account for neural status in interpretation
Can evaulate neural status	
Can use as an indirect method to estimate hearing sensitivity	Responses near thresholds may be difficult to distinguish
Can test each ear individually	Adequate neural function is necessary to use to estimate hearing status
Frequency specific and rapid recording methods available	Infant must be quiet
Not affected by sedation or sleep	Not a test of true hearing
Provides a physiological cross-check with behavioral information	May take more technical expertise and time than some other newborn screening tests

methods, such as maximum length sequences and steady state responses, allow rapid acquisition of responses.

One little-appreciated advantage over behavioral tests limited to sound-field evaluation is the ABR's ability to test each ear individually and to use both air- and bone-conducted stimuli. Isolation of individual ear responses in bone-conduction testing and in cases of asymmetric hearing is possible with the use of masking.

7.4.3.2. Limitations

The ABR does not truly assess hearing in the global sense. Absence of an ABR alone cannot be interpreted as an infallible index of severe peripheral hearing loss. This type of overinterpretation of results neglects several possibilities, only one of which is nervous system immaturity and concomitantly poor neural synchrony.

Neural status must be taken into account. Conditions such as fourth ventricle hydrocephalus and other conditions that may affect function of the eighth nerve and/or brainstem may limit the ability to use the ABR to obtain estimates of hearing sensitivity in these patients.

Even when using tonebursts or other frequency-specific stimuli, the rapid rise time necessary for synchronous discharge compromises frequency specificity at high intensities. This lack of frequency specificity may limit the ability to relate results to specific behavioral audiometric thresholds.

Distinguishing waveforms from noise at low intensities is often subjective, and criteria vary from examiner to examiner. Thus, the ABR is an objective measure in the sense that the subject need not voluntarily participate, but there is a subjective component in test interpretation.

When used to obtain information about hearing sensitivity, the ABR can be time-consuming. When testing is performed on sedated infants and children, time must be used efficiently to minimize time under sedation and to ensure that as much data as possible are obtained before the patient awakens.

7.5. NEWBORN HEARING SCREENING USING THE ABR

Historically, hearing screening programs for newborns have used ABR as a measure that provides objective information, and results are considered reliable (Cox, Hack, & Metz, 1981; Galambos & Hecox, 1978; Galambos, Hicks, & Wilson, 1982, 1984; Jacobson & Morehouse, 1984). Schulman-Galambos and Galambos (1979) reported that an effective screening program can be carried out if survivors of neonatal intensive care units are the target population.

Presently, newborn hearing screening, either universally applied to all newborns or restricted to high-risk populations, is becoming more and more prevalent, with a number of states in the United States enacting legislation in support of universal or high-risk screening performed using objective physiological techniques. The tests of choice in newborn screening programs generally are otoacoustic emissions and/or the ABR. The unique characteristics of otoacoustic emissions and ABRs provide different ways of evaluating hearing in infants. Otoacoustic emissions can be rapidly recorded and provide information about presence or absence of hearing loss, but cannot provide information about the degree or type of hearing loss. Automated ABRs also provide an efficient method of hearing screening. ABRs, with the use of frequency-specific and bone-conducted stimuli, can provide information necessary to initiate appropriate management. Currently, both otoacoustic emissions and ABRs are in widespread use and are supported by the literature and clinical practice as excellent methods of screening for hearing loss in newborns.

The role of the ABR in newborn screening programs generally is either as an initial screening technique or as the follow-up procedure used to quantify hearing sensitivity of each ear and provide information for implementation of appropriate management strategies.

One key to obtaining valid ABR results in newborns and infants relates to performing testing at a time when infants and the surrounding environment are reasonably quiet. Testing after feeding often ensures a relatively quiet state. Another consideration in the nursery is testing during times when there is less other activity that might produce higher ambient noise levels.

7.5.1. ABR Screening Methods

Screening ABRs are obtained by presenting click stimuli at one or two intensities to each ear individually. Test protocols are designed to provide information sufficient to classify results as either pass or fail.

Screening ABRs can be obtained by using either conventional ABR equipment where a set screening protocol is followed or by using an automated ABR device where test parameters and options are limited to those necessary to complete the screening procedure. With conventional systems, the clinician has control over the stimulus intensity, polarity, rate, and so on. With automated devices, stimulus and recording parameters are preset. Often, the selection of type of system is related to the personnel administering the infant hearing screening test.

It is common to select a screening intensity of about 35 dB nHL. This intensity level allows for the presence of some ambient noise, as in the nursery, but will also miss infants with mild hearing loss. Consistent with a screening approach, stimuli are presented to each ear until either a response is noted or a set number of sweeps are averaged together; then determination of the outcome is made. Some protocols will include a second screening level of about 75 dB nHL, which is used if a "fail" is obtained at 35 dB nHL.

A primary difference between conventional and screening devices relates to test interpretation. Conventional ABR devices generate waveforms that the clinician then interprets to determine the presence or absence of a response. Automated ABRs depend on an internal algorithm that compares incoming data to a statistical metric in order to internally determine whether a response is present. The automated system user is provided with a "pass" or "fail" indication, although some automated screening devices store the waveforms so that they can be retrieved and reviewed. Comparisons of outcomes with conventional and screening ABR systems generally have shown consistent results (e.g., Jacobson, Jacobson, & Spahr, 1990).

Automated ABR methods minimize the decision-making process and can sometimes be administered by individuals with minimal training. Application of electrodes, positioning of the earphones, maintenance of an acceptable test environment, and a quiet infant are all factors that are critical to the success of the screening test.

7.5.2. Retrospective Studies of ABR Testing in Newborns

Galambos et al. (1982) reviewed results on 890 babies who were screened for hearing loss using the ABR when they left a neonatal intensive care nursery. Results indicated that 10% of babies who are at risk for hearing loss may leave the hospital with reduced hearing sensitivity in one or both ears and that at least 2% may have a hearing loss severe enough to require hearing aids. In a more recent summary of 4,374 infants tested, Galambos, Wilson, and Silva (1994) reported that screening at 30 dB nHL resulted in failure rates (for one or both ears) of 19.8% for third-level intensive care nursery graduates and 12% for second-level intensive care nursery graduates. Upon return for retest, 48.7% and 44%, respectively, responded to 25-dB nHL clicks and were judged normal. Ultimately, the number of infants fitted with hearing aids were 2.1% and 1.4% of the 4,374 infants originally tested.

Jerger, Hayes, and Jordan (1980) reviewed 167 children on whom ABR testing was performed. Agreement among ABR, immittance, and behavioral test results was usually quite good. Abnormal results in children with central nervous system involvement can be ambiguous because a peripheral hearing disorder may also exist. A normal ABR, however, can contribute valuable information. Visual or somatosensory testing is sometimes used to differentiate between general central nervous system involvement and modality-specific losses.

Berlin and Shearer (1984) reported on 800 patients who were evaluated with electrocochleography (ECochG) and/or the ABR. Follow-up showed excellent agreement with behavioral test results, with disagreement between results occurring in only 6 of 800 patients using one or both of these measures. Errors were noted in 2 patients who had rising audiograms, in 3 early cases with conductive hearing loss for whom bone conduction was not performed, and in 1 patient from an interpretation error.

It is important to have carefully controlled tests and to follow up with additional ABRs when results are abnormal. ABR findings consistent with deafness or hearing loss are occasionally seen in infants who later show normal thresholds in conventional testing (e.g., Kraus, Özdamar, Stein, & Reed, 1984; Stockard & Stockard, 1981; Worthington & Peters, 1980).

7.5.3. Special Considerations in Recording ABRs in Infants

7.5.3.1. Electrode Montages

Recommended electrode montages in infants generally are either between the high forehead (F_Z) and ears (A_1, A_2) or between the high forehead and nape of the neck (C_7). Amplitude of Wave V is greatest for these electrode montages for low- as well as high-intensity stimuli (e.g., Katbamna, Metz, Bennett, & Dokler, 1996; Sininger, 1993). Differences in electrode placement between infants and adults may be related to differences in the orientation of scalp electrodes in relation to the position of the brainstem.

When newborns and infants are tested, recording electrodes often are placed at the high forehead and mastoid areas rather than the vertex and earlobe. Placement of electrodes on infant earlobes is often difficult due to the small size of the earlobe. Placement at the high forehead avoids the fontanelle area where the skull may not be fully developed.

Jacobson and Hecox (1982) reported that a horizontal (earlobe-to-earlobe) electrode montage enhances Wave I and does not decrease the amplitude of Wave V in infants younger than 6 months. They recommended use of horizontal and vertical (vertex-to-earlobe) montages when testing infants. A derived horizontal recording can be obtained with a two-channel recording montage and use of computer subtraction of the contralateral from the ipsilateral recording. Because Wave I is present only in the ipsilateral response, it will be prominent in the derived (subtracted) response.

7.5.3.2. Number of Recording Channels

The contralaterally recorded ABR is poorly developed in newborns and young infants, so the standard two-channel montage recommended for older infants, children, and adults may not yield useful information in the contralateral recording channel. The highest amplitude ABRs in infants result from vertex (C_z) or high forehead (F_z) to ipsilateral ear, or from C_z or F_z to the nape of the neck at the seventh cervical vertebrae (C_7) recording montages (Katbamna et al., 1996). Thus either a single ipsilateral channel can be used or, as some recommend, a two channel recording using F_z-ipsilateral ear and F_z–C_7 may be useful in maximizing Waves I and V. Wave I may be greatest for the F_z-ipsilateral ear montage, whereas Wave V amplitude is maximized with the F_z–C_7 montage.

7.5.3.3. Filter Characteristics

When testing infants, lowering the low-frequency filter setting from 100 Hz to 30 Hz enhances the amplitude of Wave V and improves the signal-to-noise ratio in infant ABRs (Sininger, 1995; Spivak, 1993; Stuart & Yang, 1994). Studies show that use of a 30-Hz low-frequency (high-pass) filter cutoff is preferred for both air- and bone-conducted stimuli (Stuart & Yang, 1994). The lower frequency filter cutoff yields higher amplitude ABRs because there is greater energy in the lower frequencies (below 150 Hz) in infant than adult ABRs.

Decreasing the low-frequency filter setting to 30 Hz may allow greater interference from 60-Hz electrical noise. Good electrode impedance and careful placement of electrode cables should reduce this problem. Although line noise may be a factor, the notch filter that, when activated, rejects input around 60 Hz should not be used.

7.5.3.4. Bone-Conduction ABRs in Infants

A comparison of air- and bone-conducted stimuli in premature neonates indicated a significantly greater number of detectable bone- than air-conduction responses, which suggests that a combination of the two be used (Hooks &

Weber, 1984). Use of bone-conduction stimuli may decrease the problem of failures due to transient middle ear problems, which Jacobson and Morehouse (1984) showed to be present in 44% of their failures, as well as due to collapsed ear canals (Hosford-Dunn, Runge, Hillel, & Johnson, 1983). In another study of high-risk infants, the failure rate for air-conducted clicks was reported as 20.6% and two thirds of these failures were found to be conductive in nature (Yang, Stuart, Mencher et al., 1993). Reliable bone-conduction ABRs can be recorded in infants (Yang, Stuart, Stenstrom, & Green, 1993) and the findings of these studies underscore the importance of including bone-conduction ABR testing when the ABR is used to estimate hearing sensitivity.

An important consideration in bone conduction testing in infants is stimulus intensity level differences between infants and adults. Skull differences between infants and adults, resulting in higher intensity levels at the cochlea, may account for latency, amplitude, and threshold differences (Cone-Wesson & Ramirez, 1997; Foxe & Stapells, 1993; Stuart, Yang, & Stenstrom, 1990; Yang, Rupert, & Moushegian, 1987). Smaller temporal bone size relative to the oscillator and lack of ossification of temporal bone sutures also could contribute to these differences.

Middle ear status in newborns clearly affects otoacoustic emissions and may also affect ABR thresholds. Cochlear sensitivity may be better than thresholds obtained using air-conducted stimuli due either to debris remaining in the external ear canal or middle ear space in newborns or to transient middle ear pathology in infants and children. Bone-conducted stimuli provide a method of overcoming external and middle ear effects and may be useful as a screening tool.

7.5.3.5. Waveform Interpretation and Normative Data

Stockard and Stockard (1981) suggested that recording Wave I (the surface-recorded eighth nerve action potential) and Wave V provides a practical and effective screening method. Wave I has been reported to be a more precise index of middle ear (Mendelson et al., 1979) and inner ear (Coats & Martin, 1977) function because it is unaffected by more central abnormalities. Weber (1982) suggested the use of norms that utilize the Wave III or Waves I–III interval as the indicator of brainstem maturation in infants, because earlier components may be more sensitive than conventional normative values based on Wave V.

In patients older than 18 months, adult normative data generally can be used in interpretation. In infants, we expect increased absolute and interwave latencies (see Figure 7–3) and use normative data adapted from the data of Zimmerman et al. (1987). A Wave V latency-intensity function for air-conduction clicks including ± three standard deviations is shown in Figure 7–3. Infant and adult Wave V latency-intensity functions, including ± 3 standard deviation ranges, are compared in Figure 7–4.

The latency differences between infants and adults are less for low-frequency stimuli than for clicks. Thus, prolongations in latency over adult values are ex-

LATENCY-INTENSITY FUNCTION FOR INFANTS

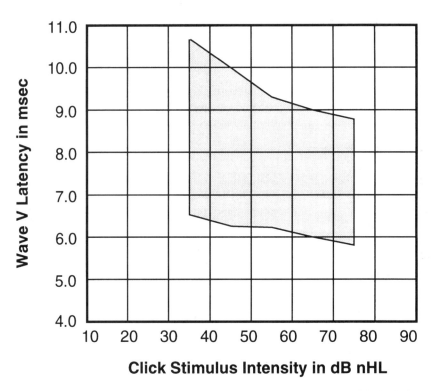

Figure 7–3. Normal ABR Wave V latency-intensity function for infants for clicks showing a range of ±3 standard deviations. (Adapted from data from "Auditory Brain Stem Evoked Response Characteristics in Developing Infants," by M. C. Zimmerman, D. E. Morgan, and J. R. Dubno, 1987, *Annals of Otology, Rhinology and Laryngology, 96,* pp. 291–299.)

pected for low-frequency tonebursts, but not to the same degree as when comparing clicks.

7.5.3.6. Ear and Gender Differences in the ABR

Gender differences are apparent in infant ABRs as well as adult ABRs. Female infants exhibit shorter latencies, higher amplitude responses, and lower thresholds for air-conducted clicks and tonebursts (Eldredge & Salamy, 1996; Hyde, Matsumoto, & Alberti, 1987). Small but significant ear differences also have been reported, which are characterized by higher amplitude and shorter interwave latency intervals (Eldredge & Salamy, 1996). Cone-Wesson and Ramirez (1997)

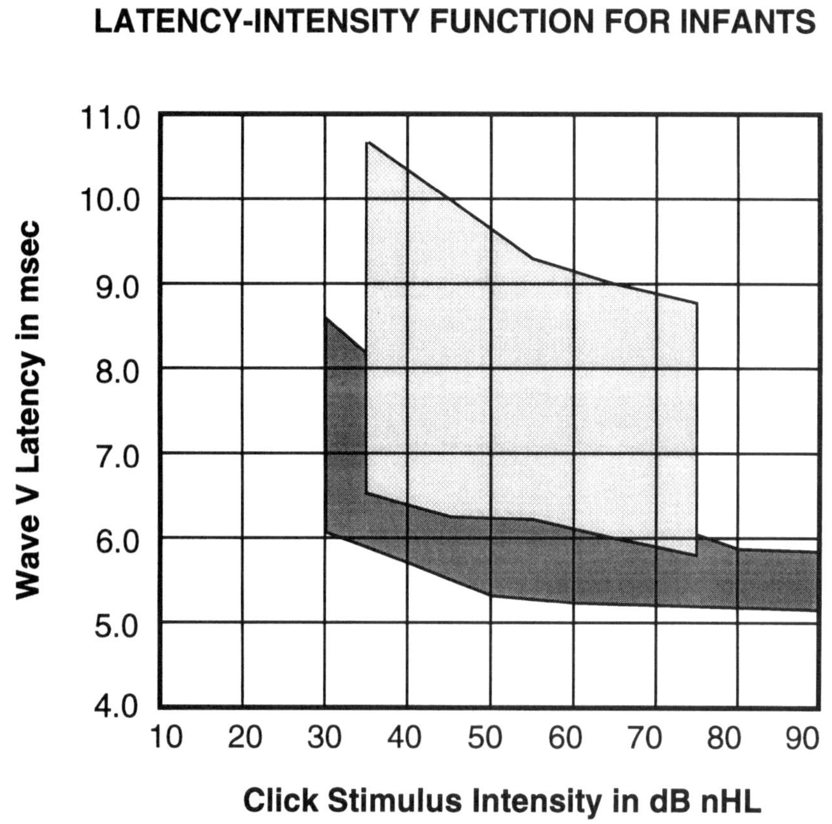

LATENCY-INTENSITY FUNCTION FOR INFANTS

Figure 7-4. Comparison of infant and adult Wave V latency-intensity functions for clicks. The adult latency-intensity function is shown in dark gray and the infant latency-intensity function is shown in light gray.

reported that bone-conducted ABRs in newborns also show lower thresholds in females than males.

7.5.3.7. Relation Between ABR Thresholds and Behavioral Thresholds

The lowest intensity levels where ABRs are observed for air-conducted stimuli are reported to be higher in neonates than adults when intensity levels are monitored in the ear canal (Schulman-Galambos & Galambos, 1979; Sininger, Abdala, & Cone-Wesson, 1997). Differences range from approximately 5 to 25 dB, and greater differences are reported for higher frequency stimuli. The gap between neonatal and adult thresholds appears to close by about 24 months of age. Differences in characteristics between neonate and adult ear canals and errors in estimation when coupler calibration is used may contribute to the discrepancy. Monitoring of stimulus levels in the ear canal with a probe microphone should allow accurate determination of actual response threshold levels.

Cone-Wesson and Ramirez (1997) measured sound pressure levels of bone-conducted stimuli in the ear canal and found that infant bone-conduction ABR thresholds were in fairly good agreement with adult thresholds for stimuli centered at 500 Hz but showed a greater difference at 4000 Hz, which is in agreement with air-conduction findings.

ABR thresholds for tonebursts (centered at 500, 2000, and 4000 Hz) in notched noise show quite good agreement with behavioral thresholds in infants and young children with normal hearing and with cochlear hearing loss (Stapells et al., 1995). Overall, 93% of the children showed agreement within 20 dB between ABR and behavioral thresholds, and 80% were within 15 dB. ABR thresholds for 500-Hz tonebursts were about 10 dB higher than for the other frequencies evaluated.

7.6. AUDITORY NEUROPATHY IN INFANTS AND YOUNG CHILDREN

The evaluation of patients with an auditory neuropathy provides an excellent example of the rationale for use of a test battery approach to audiological evaluation. In the instance of infants and young children, physiological tests are particularly valuable because they are objective and are uniquely suited to identify auditory neuropathy. The three measures discussed in this chapter, otoacoustic emissions, MEMRs, and ABR, are the most powerful methods available to discriminate an auditory neuropathy from other auditory disorders.

The term *auditory neuropathy,* as discussed in Chapter 5, describes patients who demonstrate normal otoacoustic emissions and absent or grossly abnormal ABRs (e.g., Berlin et al., 1993, 1994; Starr et al., 1991, 1996). The normal otoacoustic emissions suggest normal outer hair cell function, and the abnormal ABRs are consistent with a neural disorder.

Patients with an auditory neuropathy are readily identifiable clinically, and of particular interest to pediatric evaluation is the fact that infants and young children have been identified with auditory neuropathy (Berlin et al., 1998; Stein et al., 1996). As discussed earlier, infants and children in particular may show ABRs that *seem* to have repeatable responses. However, on close examination, it is found that the latency of the responses does not increase with decreasing intensity, as should occur with neural responses. When polarity of the stimulus (i.e., changing from condensation to rarefaction clicks) is reversed, the recorded responses also reverse, which is characteristic of cochlear microphonics rather than an ABR.

Management strategies for infants and young children with an auditory neuropathy are particularly critical to the development of language. Berlin et al. (1998)

encourage the use of Cued Speech or other methods that introduce visual information that follows the structure of English, because some of them may "outgrow" their neuropathy and later be able to use the cue-supported auditory information in a normal manner. The probability of this is simply not known at the present time, but the importance of management for all children with an auditory neuropathy lies in facilitating development of language and communication skills.

Older patients with auditory neuropathy generally have *not* found amplification helpful, which is expected in view of their normal otoacoustic emissions; however, some children with auditory neuropathy have used hearing aids and a few children have been managed with cochlear implants. Success in learning language using a purely auditory mode is questionable unless the neuropathy is not due to neural dyssynchrony or the dyssynchrony resolves.

PART III

Case Studies and Report Writing

ABR Case Studies

The auditory brainstem response (ABR) should be considered only one component of a battery of test measures. A reasonable conclusion regarding auditory function and/or the nature of a disorder should be obtained through comparison of the results of several measures of auditory function and other evaluations appropriate to the suspected problem.

As with any diagnostic procedure, the importance of obtaining thorough case history information cannot be overemphasized. Information about medical conditions, medications, and results of other medical tests should be obtained. Audiometric data are essential in appropriate interpretation of test results and, in most cases, patient management following ABR evaluation. Current audiometric data pertaining to air- and bone-conduction sensitivity should be obtained in all cases where patients can be tested behaviorally. Evaluation of middle ear function, including tympanograms and ipsilateral and contralateral middle ear muscle reflexes (MEMRs), is particularly useful in testing infants and young children, but should be applied to the evaluation of all patients, to rule out middle ear disorders.

Several studies have compared the results of MEMR levels, reflex decay measures, and the results of the ABR. Excellent agreement has been reported between these measures in distinguishing cochlear and retrocochlear sites, and they serve as a reliable cross-check (Hayes & Jerger, 1981). Abnormal middle ear function and prolonged absolute latency of all waveforms are consistent with the presence of a conductive or mixed hearing loss. Absent MEMRs with no middle ear abnormality and a prolonged or absent ABR may suggest a sensory or neural hearing loss, depending on the pure-tone sensitivity and, in some cases, the presence or absence of otoacoustic emissions.

In the following case studies, summarized in Table 8–1, audiometric, middle ear, and auditory evoked potential findings are presented along with other measures appropriate to the evaluation of the particular patients. The key to audiometric symbols is shown in Table 8–2.

8.1. CASE STUDY 1: UNILATERAL COCHLEAR HEARING LOSS AND A NORMAL ABR

HISTORY

This patient is a 14-year-old female who was referred for audiological evaluation following failure of a hearing test at school. Her family was unaware of a hearing problem, although they did report that she frequently asked for repetition of conversation. Birth and developmental history were unremarkable.

Table 8-1. Summary of ABR case studies.

Cochlear Hearing Loss and Normal ABR

Case Study 1	Unilateral cochlear hearing loss
Case Study 2	High-frequency asymmetric cochlear hearing loss
Case Study 3	Cochlear hearing loss, abnormal summating potential

Eighth Nerve/Brainstem Lesions

Case Study 4	Adult with normal hearing and eighth nerve tumor
Case Study 5	Adult with asymmetric hearing loss and eighth nerve tumor
Case Study 6	Adult with asymmetric hearing loss and eighth nerve tumor
Case Study 7	Adult with eighth nerve tumor and abnormal rate effect
Case Study 8	Adult with unilateral hearing loss and eighth nerve tumor
Case Study 9	Adult with meningioma
Case Study 10	Adult with brainstem gliomas

Estimation of Hearing Sensitivity

Case Study 11	Infant with normal hearing
Case Study 12	Child with a bilateral conductive hearing loss
Case Study 13	Child with unilateral atresia
Case Study 14	Child with a moderate sensory hearing loss
Case Study 15	Child with a unilateral sensory hearing loss

Auditory Neuropathy

Case Study 16	Adult with an auditory neuropathy
Case Study 17	Infant with an auditory neuropathy

Technical Errors

Case Study 18	Collapsed ear canal
Case Study 19	Postauricular muscle artifact
Case Study 20	Erroneous electrode connection

Table 8-2. Key to audiometric symbols.

Test Condition	Right Ear	Both Ears	Left Ear
Air conduction			
Unmasked	O		X
Masked	△		☐
Bone conduction (mastoid)			
Unmasked	<		>
Masked	[		]
Bone conduction (forehead)			
Unmasked		V	
Masked	˥		⌐
No response	↘		↙
Absent	Ab		Ab

AUDIOMETRIC TEST RESULTS

Pure-tone audiometry indicated normal hearing thresholds in the right ear and a mild to moderate sensory hearing loss in the left ear. Speech reception thresholds were consistent with pure-tone results. Speech recognition in quiet for monosyllables was normal for the right ear (100% at 40 dB HL) and significantly reduced for the left ear (56% at 70 dB HL). Speech recognition at higher intensities in quiet for the left ear was 56% at 80 dB HL and 64% at 90 dB HL. Loudness balance testing was consistent with recruitment in the left ear. Pure-tone and speech Stenger tests were negative. Audiometric test results are shown in Figure 8–1.

MIDDLE EAR TEST RESULTS

Middle ear testing showed normal tympanograms bilaterally. Contralateral MEMR thresholds were normal in the right ear and elevated in the higher frequencies in the left ear. Reflex decay was negative for each ear.

ABR RESULTS

Evoked potential testing was pursued due to the presence of a unilateral sensory hearing loss and poor speech recognition ability in the left ear. ABR testing indicated normal absolute and interwave latencies for stimulation of the right and left ears at 85 dB nHL and a click rate of 7.7 stimuli per second. ABRs obtained at click rates of 27.7 and 57.7 per second were also normal. Wave V was symmetric between ears. Wave I latency was longer in the left than right ear, resulting in a shortened Waves I–V interwave interval in the left ear. The ABR results are shown in Figure 8–2.

OUTCOME

Normal ABR, consistent with a cochlear hearing loss.

COMMENT

This case demonstrates a normal ABR with a cochlear hearing loss and a similarity between responses obtained for the normal and affected ears when stimuli are presented at high intensities. No correction factor is required and, in fact, the latency of Wave V is shorter in the ear with the hearing loss, resulting in a shorter Waves I–V interval in that ear. A shortened Waves I–V interval is sometimes observed in cochlear hearing loss. When hearing thresholds in the higher frequencies are better than approximately 60 dB HL, a normal ABR should be anticipated if the loss is cochlear in origin. This case also is instructive in that, when using the ABR to estimate hearing sensitivity, presentation of stimuli at a single high-intensity would miss a significant hearing loss such as this one.

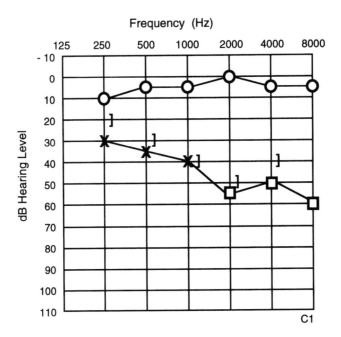

PURE TONE THRESHOLDS

MIDDLE EAR MUSCLE REFLEXES

((😊 Stimulus Right					😊)) Stimulus Left				
	500	1k	2k	4k		500	1k	2k	4k
Contra	80	80	90	85	Contra	85	95	Ab	Ab
Ipsi	DNT	DNT	DNT	DNT	Ipsi	DNT	DNT	DNT	DNT

SPEECH AUDIOMETRY

Test Condition	Right Ear	Left Ear
Words in Quiet (PB Max)	100% at 40 HL	56% at 70 HL 64% at 90 HL

Figure 8-1. Audiometric test results for Case Study 1.

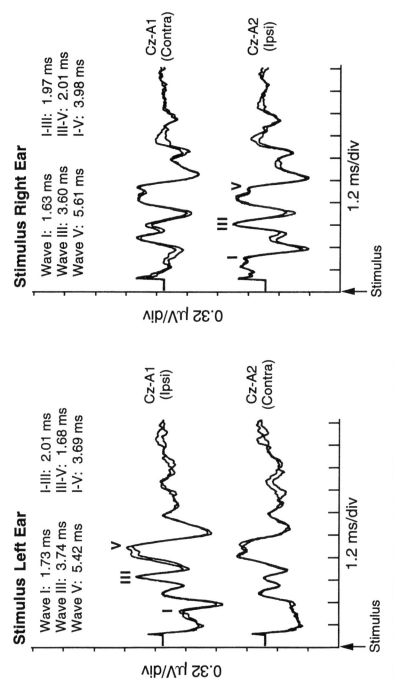

Stimulus Right Ear

Wave I: 1.63 ms   I-III: 1.97 ms
Wave III: 3.60 ms   III-V: 2.01 ms
Wave V: 5.61 ms   I-V: 3.98 ms

Cz-A1 (Contra)

Cz-A2 (Ipsi)

0.32 µV/div

1.2 ms/div

Stimulus

Stimulus Left Ear

Wave I: 1.73 ms   I-III: 2.01 ms
Wave III: 3.74 ms   III-V: 1.68 ms
Wave V: 5.42 ms   I-V: 3.69 ms

Cz-A1 (Ipsi)

Cz-A2 (Contra)

0.32 µV/div

1.2 ms/div

Stimulus

Figure 8–2. ABR results for clicks at 7.7 per second for Case Study 1.

8.2. CASE STUDY 2: HIGH-FREQUENCY ASYMMETRIC COCHLEAR HEARING LOSS

HISTORY

This patient is a 54-year-old male who reported a hearing loss, greater in the left ear, which decreased following an incident of assault 7 months prior to the current evaluation. He also reported bilateral tinnitus that was worse in the left ear and occasional exposure to loud music, but no other significant noise exposure.

AUDIOMETRIC TEST RESULTS

Pure-tone audiometry indicated a mild to moderate high-frequency hearing loss of the configuration associated with a noise-induced hearing loss in the right ear and a severe high-frequency hearing loss in the left ear. Speech thresholds were consistent with pure-tone results and a pure-tone Stenger test was negative. Word recognition was normal in the right ear and reduced (36% at 50 dB HL and 60% at 80 dB HL) in the left ear. Transient evoked and distortion product otoacoustic emissions were present and consistent with a high-frequency hearing loss bilaterally. Audiometric and otoacoustic emission test results are shown in Figures 8–3 and 8–4, respectively.

MIDDLE EAR TEST RESULTS

Middle ear testing indicated tympanograms within the normal range and normal ipsilateral and contralateral MEMR thresholds with the exception of stimulation of the left ear at 4000 Hz.

ABR RESULTS

ABR testing was indicated based on the asymmetric hearing loss and history. ABRs were obtained with clicks presented at 7.7, 27.7, and 57.7 stimuli per second and intensity levels of 90 dB nHL for the right ear and 90 and 95 dB nHL for the left ear. Simultaneous presentation of clicks at 90 dB nHL in the right ear and 95 dB nHL resulted in behavioral midline localization of the stimulus. Responses to condensation and rarefaction clicks were both within the normal range. Responses for the right and left ears were within normal limits for absolute and interwave latencies as well as for Waves V/I amplitude comparisons. Latency increases with increasing stimulus presentation rate were within the normal range. The ABR results are shown in Figure 8–5.

OUTCOME

Normal ABR, consistent with a cochlear hearing loss.

PURE TONE THRESHOLDS

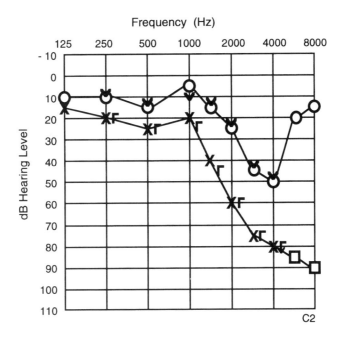

MIDDLE EAR MUSCLE REFLEXES

	Stimulus Right					Stimulus Left			
	500	1k	2k	4k		500	1k	2k	4k
Contra	90	85	85	90	Contra	85	90	90	Ab
Ipsi	75	80	80	90	Ipsi	80	80	80	100

SPEECH AUDIOMETRY

Test Condition	Right Ear	Left Ear
PB Words in Quiet	92% at 50 HL	36% at 50 HL 60% at 80 HL

Figure 8-3. Audiometric test results for Case Study 2.

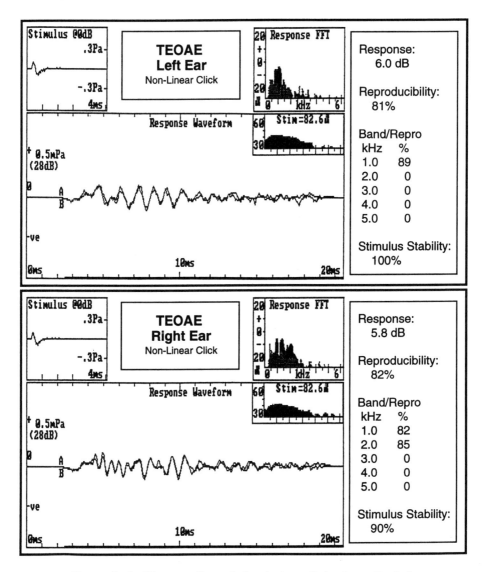

Figure 8-4. Otoacoustic emission test results for Case Study 2.

COMMENT

The ABR obtained with stimulation of the right ear is much clearer than the ABR from the left ear. Although morphology was quite different, responses in both ears met the criteria for a normal ABR: replicability, normal absolute latencies, normal interwave latencies, normal amplitude relationship between Waves I and V, and a normal increase in latency with increased presentation rate. Responses obtained for the right and left ears were compared both at equal intensity levels (90 dB nHL) and at intensities where the clicks localized behaviorally to the midline. Sometimes comparison of responses at levels where the clicks midline

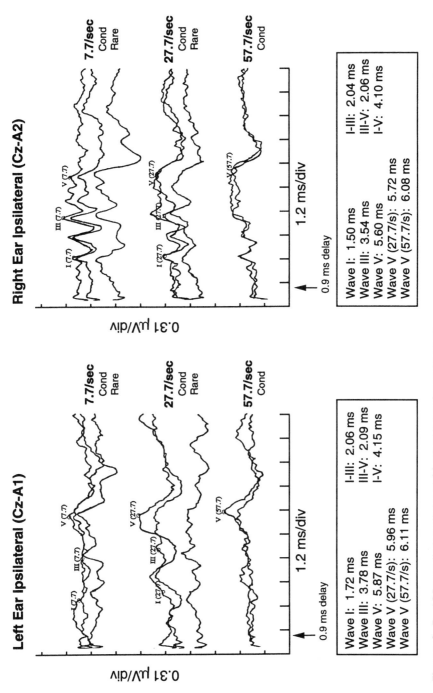

Figure 8–5. ABR results for clicks at 90 dB nHL for Case Study 2.

localize is helpful in cases with asymmetric hearing loss. In this patient, responses were within the normal range for all intensities. No correction for hearing loss was necessary.

8.3. CASE STUDY 3: COCHLEAR HEARING LOSS WITH A NEGATIVE SUMMATING POTENTIAL

HISTORY

This patient is a 62-year-old female who reported a progressive hearing loss, headaches, and occasional dizziness. Case history also indicated high blood pressure and diabetes.

AUDIOMETRIC TEST RESULTS

Pure-tone audiometry showed essentially normal hearing in the right ear and a mild to moderate hearing loss in the left ear, with the poorest hearing in the lower frequencies. Word recognition was very poor (20% at 80 dB HL) in the left ear. Audiometric test results are shown in Figure 8–6.

MIDDLE EAR TEST RESULTS

Tympanograms were normal bilaterally, and contralateral MEMRs were present and symmetric, although slightly elevated in each ear for the frequencies of 500, 1000, and 2000 Hz.

ABR RESULTS

This patient was referred for ABR testing on the basis of case history complaints and poor speech recognition in the left ear to rule out the presence of a retro-cochlear disorder. ABRs to clicks presented at 85 dB nHL and 27.7 stimuli per second showed normal absolute and interwave latencies for the right and left ears. The ABR results are shown in Figure 8–7.

INTERPRETATION

Normal ABR. Comparison of the ipsilateral responses in the right and left ears showed a negative summating potential (see arrow on Figure 8–7) for the left ear response. This finding is considered consistent with Ménière's disease (Coats, 1981).

COMMENT

In this case the ABR was useful in both ruling out a retrocochlear disorder and assisting in the diagnosis of the type of cochlear disorder. Testing with insert earphones, an ear canal electrode, or transtympanic electrocochleography (ECochG) may be used to further define the cochlear response.

PURE TONE THRESHOLDS

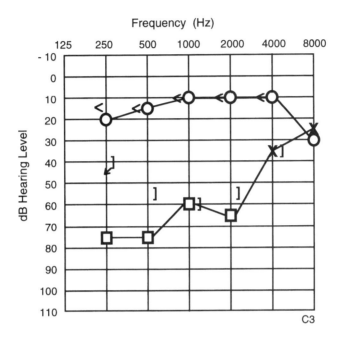

MIDDLE EAR MUSCLE REFLEXES

(◖ ☺) Stimulus Right				(☺)◗ Stimulus Left			
	500	1k	2k	4k	500	1k	2k	4k
Contra	95	90	100	Ab	Contra 100	90	95	Ab
Ipsi	DNT	DNT	DNT	DNT	Ipsi DNT	DNT	DNT	DNT

SPEECH AUDIOMETRY

Test Condition	Right Ear	Left Ear
Words in Quiet (PB Max)	100% at 55 HL	20% at 80 HL

Figure 8-6. Audiometric test results for Case Study 3.

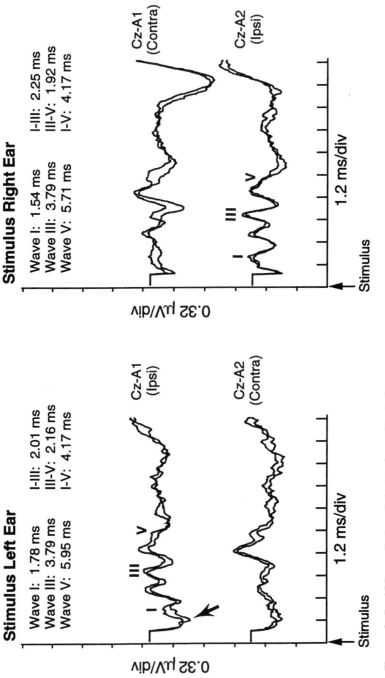

Figure 8–7. ABR results for clicks for Case Study 3.

8.4. CASE STUDY 4: ADULT WITH HEARING WITHIN NORMAL LIMITS AND AN EIGHTH NERVE TUMOR

HISTORY

This patient is a 33-year-old female who was seen for routine evaluation in a hospital outpatient otology clinic with a complaint of dizziness but no noticeable hearing loss.

AUDIOMETRIC TEST RESULTS

Pure-tone audiometry indicated hearing thresholds within the normal range bilaterally and speech recognition in quiet within normal limits for each ear. A slight asymmetry in thresholds was noted. Further audiological testing indicated poor speech recognition in noise (56% at 55 dB HL with a +10 signal-to-noise ratio) and positive PIPB rollover (to 52% at 70 dB HL) for speech presented to the right ear. Audiometric test results are shown in Figure 8–8.

MIDDLE EAR TEST RESULTS

Tympanograms were consistent with normal middle ear function. Ipsilateral and contralateral MEMRs were elevated for the right ear, and reflex decay was positive in that ear.

ABR RESULTS

The patient was referred for ABR evaluation based on the abnormal MEMRs and poor speech recognition ability. The ABR for the left ear showed normal absolute and interwave latencies for stimuli presented at 85 dB nHL at a rate of 27.7 clicks per second. Results for the right ear indicated normal latency for Wave I and prolonged latencies for Waves III and V and the I–III and I–V interwave intervals. The ABR results are shown in Figure 8–9.

OTHER TEST RESULTS

Computed tomography (CT) showed a mass measuring 1.28 cm in the coronal and sagittal planes adjacent to the internal auditory canal on the right. Vestibular testing showed right unilateral weakness (56%) and left directional preponderance (31%) with no spontaneous or positional nystagmus.

OUTCOME

Surgery was performed using a translabyrinthine approach, which resulted in removal of an extracanicular cerebellar pontine angle tumor with preservation of

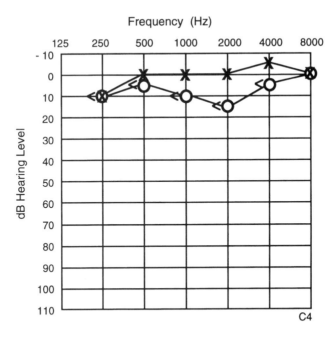

Figure 8–8. Audiometric test results for Case Study 4.

the eighth nerve. No measurable hearing was preserved in the right ear post-surgically. The pathology report indicated a 1.2-cm benign neurilemmoma.

COMMENT

This case is particularly instructive in that routine pure-tone audiometry and speech audiometry in quiet were normal for both ears, although there was a very

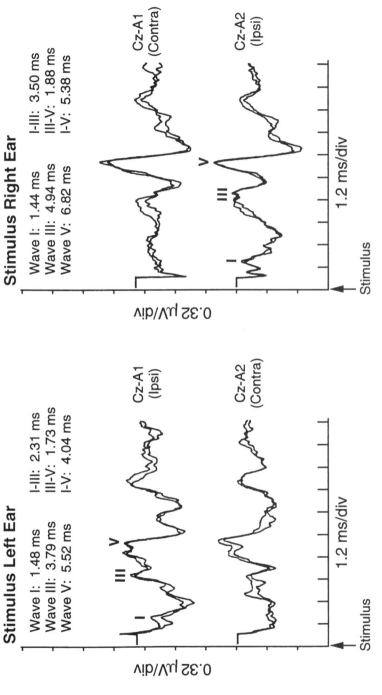

Figure 8–9. ABR results for clicks for Case Study 4.

subtle asymmetry between ears in pure-tone thresholds. The first indication of a possible abnormality in the auditory system was the abnormal MEMRs. This case demonstrates the importance of using the unexplained MEMR abnormality as a reason to obtain an ABR and shows that at least one type of objective physiological measure should be an essential component of all evaluations.

8.5. CASE STUDY 5: ADULT WITH ASYMMETRIC HEARING LOSS AND AN EIGHTH NERVE TUMOR

HISTORY

This patient is a 70-year-old female who reported a history of allergies, a change in her hearing over the 6 months prior to the hearing test, no dizziness, and no other medical problems or symptoms.

AUDIOMETRIC TEST RESULTS

Pure-tone audiometry indicated an asymmetric sloping sensorineural hearing loss with poorer hearing in the right ear. Speech thresholds were consistent with

pure-tone results. Word recognition in quiet was excellent (100% at 55 dB HL) in the left ear and reduced (60% at 75 dB HL) in the right ear. PIPB rollover was noted for the right ear, with word recognition decreasing to 32% at 85 dB HL. These test results are shown in Figure 8–10.

MIDDLE EAR TEST RESULTS

Middle ear immittance showed normal middle ear compliance and slight negative pressure (-50 mm) in the left ear. Contralateral MEMRs were normal for the left ear and elevated for the right ear. Ipsilateral MEMRs were in the high-normal range and symmetric between ears. Reflex decay was positive in the right ear.

ABR RESULTS

ABRs showed Waves I, III, and V for both ears. Absolute and interwave latencies were normal in the left ear. The right ear showed a normal absolute latency for Wave I and delayed absolute latencies for Waves III and V, resulting in prolonged I–III and I–V interwave intervals. The ABR results are shown in Figure 8–11.

OTHER TEST RESULTS

Electronystagmography showed a right reduced response on caloric testing and no spontaneous or gaze nystagmus. CT scans with and without contrast (ob-

PURE TONE THRESHOLDS

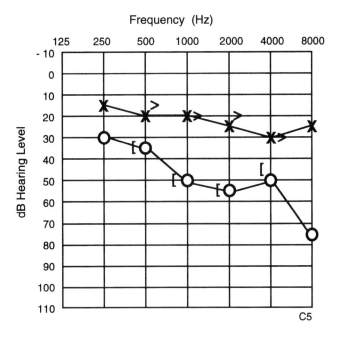

MIDDLE EAR MUSCLE REFLEXES

(•(☺) Stimulus Right				(☺)•) Stimulus Left			
	500	1k	2k	4k	500	1k	2k	4k
Contra	105	100	100	Ab	Contra	85	90	95	90
Ipsi	DNT	95	90	DNT	Ipsi	DNT	95	90	DNT

SPEECH AUDIOMETRY

Test Condition	Right Ear	Left Ear
Words in Quiet (PB Max) Words at High Intensity	60% at 75 HL 32% at 85 HL	100% at 55 HL

Figure 8-10. Audiometric test results for Case Study 5.

tained in 1983) were reported negative. An air-contrast cysternagram, obtained a few months later, revealed an intracanicular acoustic neuroma filling two thirds of the internal auditory meatus (5-mm diameter, 8-mm length).

OUTCOME

A small vestibular schwannoma was removed from the right eighth nerve.

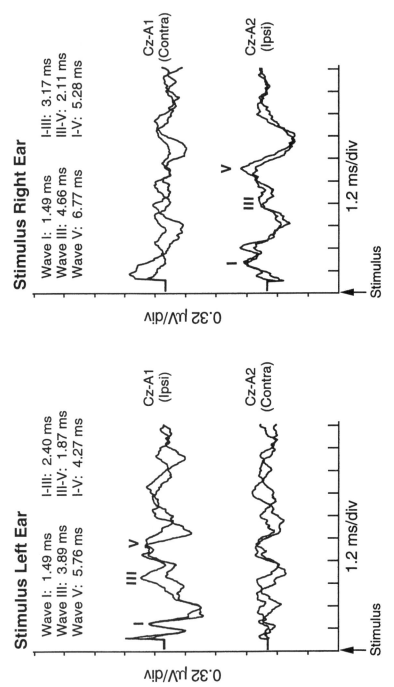

Figure 8–11. ABR results for clicks for Case Study 5. Stimulus rate was 7.7 clicks per second, and stimulus intensity was 85 dB nHL.

COMMENT

Small eighth nerve tumors (less than 1.5 cm) are often missed by CT scan, which was the standard for radiological testing at the time this patient was seen. Presently, magnetic resonance imaging (MRI) is able to distinguish many of these small tumors. This patient's ABR on the affected side presented some interpretation difficulty related to identification of Wave I. However, with hearing thresholds in the higher frequencies better than 55 dB HL, a normal ABR would be expected if the loss were cochlear in origin (see Case Study 1).

8.6. CASE STUDY 6: ADULT WITH ASYMMETRIC HEARING LOSS AND AN EIGHTH NERVE TUMOR

HISTORY

This patient is a 57-year-old female who was referred for an ABR due to asymmetric hearing loss and abnormal MEMRs. She reported a history of gradual hearing loss over approximately 15 years, with a noticeable decrease in the left ear over the past few months, ear infections, bilateral tinnitus, difficulty understanding speech, and occasional headaches. No dizziness or balance problems were reported.

AUDIOMETRIC TEST RESULTS

Pure-tone audiometry indicated a moderate high-frequency hearing loss in the right ear and a moderate to severe sensorineural hearing loss in the left ear. Speech thresholds were consistent with pure-tone results. Word recognition was normal in the right ear and reduced (60% at 80 dB HL) in the left ear. Evoked otoacoustic emissions were consistent with a high-frequency hearing loss in the right ear and were absent in the left ear. Audiometric and otoacoustic emission test results are shown in Figures 8–12 and 8–13, respectively.

MIDDLE EAR TEST RESULTS

Middle ear testing indicated normal tympanograms bilaterally. MEMRs were normal on stimulation of the right ear and absent on stimulation of the left ear.

ABR RESULTS

ABRs were obtained with clicks presented at 7.7, 27.7, and 57.7 per second at intensity levels of 80 dB nHL for the right ear and 80, 90, and 100 dB nHL for the left ear. Absolute and interwave latencies were within normal limits for the right ear. Results for the left ear showed a large cochlear microphonic, which reversed with changes in stimulus polarity from condensation to rarefaction. Waves I and

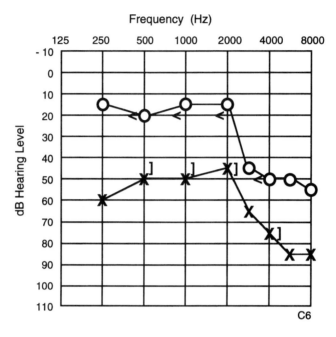

PURE TONE THRESHOLDS

MIDDLE EAR MUSCLE REFLEXES

((• Stimulus Right					Stimulus Left			
	500	1k	2k	4k		500	1k	2k	4k
Contra	100	90	85	100	Contra	Ab	Ab	Ab	Ab
Ipsi	80	90	85	85	Ipsi	Ab	Ab	Ab	Ab

SPEECH AUDIOMETRY

Test Condition	Right Ear	Left Ear
PB Words in Quiet	92% at 55 HL	60% at 80 HL

Figure 8–12. Audiometric test results for Case Study 6.

V were present with delayed absolute latency of each wave, and the Waves I–V interval was also prolonged (5.47 ms). Wave V latency increases with faster stimulus rates were within normal limits. The ABR results obtained at 80 dB nHL for each ear are shown in Figure 8–14.

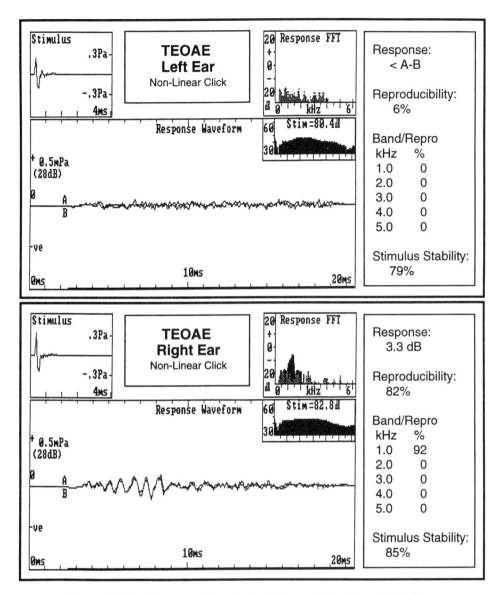

Figure 8-13. Otoacoustic emission test results for Case Study 6.

OTHER TEST RESULTS

MRI indicated a 1.5- to 2.0-cm enhancing tumor in the cerebellar pontine angle, indenting the brainstem and cerebellum, with minimal involvement of the internal auditory canal.

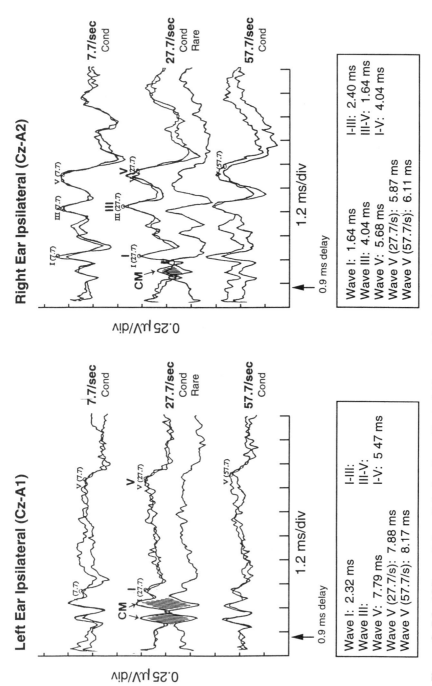

Figure 8–14. ABR results for clicks for Case Study 6. The cochlear microphonic is highlighted with shading in the middle tracings.

OUTCOME

Retrosigmoid removal of a left vestibular schwannoma. Postsurgical follow-up indicated a profound hearing loss in the left ear.

COMMENT

The prolonged Waves I–V interval was clearly abnormal and consistent with a retrocochlear lesion. This case demonstrates that comparison of responses obtained with condensation and rarefaction clicks can be useful in distinguishing cochlear and neural components. Identification of the cochlear microphonic helped to identify Wave I and determine the Waves I–V interwave latency.

8.7. CASE STUDY 7: ADULT WITH AN EIGHTH NERVE TUMOR AND AN ABNORMAL ABR RATE EFFECT

HISTORY

This patient is a 74-year-old female who reported bilateral hearing loss that was worsening in the right ear.

AUDIOMETRIC TEST RESULTS

Pure-tone audiometry indicated a moderate to severe sensorineural hearing loss in the right ear and a mild to moderate sensorineural hearing loss in the left ear. Speech thresholds were consistent with the pure-tone hearing loss. Word recognition in quiet was reduced in both ears, with poorer word recognition (44% at 90 dB HL) in the right ear. Audiometric test results are shown in Figure 8–15.

MIDDLE EAR TEST RESULTS

Middle ear testing indicated normal tympanograms bilaterally. Ipsilateral and contralateral MEMR thresholds in the left ear were normal in the lower frequencies and absent at 4000 Hz, which is consistent with the hearing loss. In the right ear, MEMR thresholds were in the high-normal range at 500 Hz and elevated or absent at all other frequencies.

ABR RESULTS

ABR testing was completed based on the asymmetric hearing loss and elevated reflex thresholds. ABRs were obtained to condensation and rarefaction clicks presented at rates of 7.7, 27.7, and 57.7 stimuli per second. Stimuli were presented at 100 dB nHL in the right ear and 85 dB nHL in the left ear. The ABR waveforms and latencies are shown in Figure 8–16. Absolute latencies were

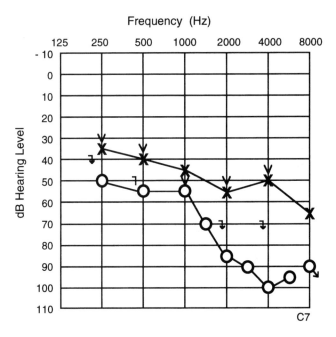

PURE TONE THRESHOLDS

MIDDLE EAR MUSCLE REFLEXES

	Stimulus Right					Stimulus Left			
	500	1k	2k	4k		500	1k	2k	4k
Contra	95	105	Ab	Ab	Contra	90	85	100	Ab
Ipsi	DNT	Ab	DNT	DNT	Ipsi	DNT	90	DNT	DNT

SPEECH AUDIOMETRY

Test Condition	Right Ear	Left Ear
PB Words in Quiet	44% at 90 HL	68% at 85 HL

Figure 8–15. Audiometric test results for Case Study 7.

longer in the right ear than the left ear, which may have been related to the greater high-frequency hearing loss in the right ear. The Waves I–III interval was at the upper limit of normal in the right ear, but suspicious because it was 0.20 ms longer for the 27.7/second rate than the Waves I–III interval obtained for the left ear.

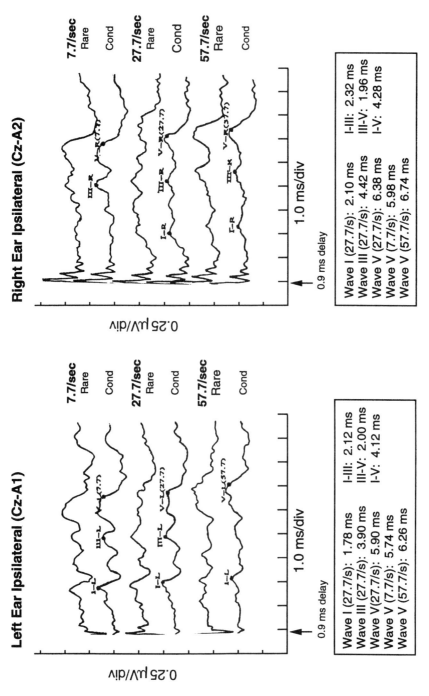

Figure 8-16. ABR results for clicks for Case Study 7.

Comparisons of increases in the absolute latencies of Wave V as a function of rate increases showed a greater effect of rate on latency in the right ear. A rate increase from 7.7 to 27.7 stimuli per second resulted in a 0.40-ms latency change (compared to 0.16 ms in the left ear) and from 7.7 to 57.7 stimuli per second showed a 0.76-ms increase (compared to 0.52 ms in the left ear). ABR results were interpreted as suspicious based on absolute and interwave latencies and abnormal latency changes with increasing stimulus rate.

OUTCOME

This patient had an intracanicular vestibular schwannoma on the right that was 12 mm in diameter.

COMMENT

This case demonstrates the importance of comparing responses obtained from each ear for symmetry. In this patient, there was an asymmetry in the length of the Waves I–III interval. Absolute latencies can be asymmetric when high-frequency hearing thresholds exceed 60 dB HL. However, interwave latencies should be symmetric if the site of the disorder is cochlear or conductive. In this patient, the interwave latency asymmetry was further supported by abnormal rate increases in the right ear and the elevated and absent MEMRs.

8.8. CASE STUDY 8: SEVERE UNILATERAL HEARING LOSS AND A VESTIBULAR SCHWANNOMA

HISTORY

This patient was referred because of a unilateral hearing loss identified by pure-tone threshold testing.

AUDIOMETRIC TEST RESULTS

Pure-tone thresholds showed a severe to profound hearing loss in the right ear and normal hearing in the left ear. A normal speech reception threshold was obtained in the left ear, and the speech awareness threshold was consistent with a severe hearing loss for the right ear. Word recognition was normal in the left ear; no words were understood in the right ear. Audiometric test results are shown in Figure 8–17.

MIDDLE EAR TEST RESULTS

Tympanograms were normal bilaterally. Ipsilateral and contralateral MEMR thresholds were normal on stimulation of the left ear. Reflexes were elevated and absent when the right ear was stimulated.

PURE TONE THRESHOLDS

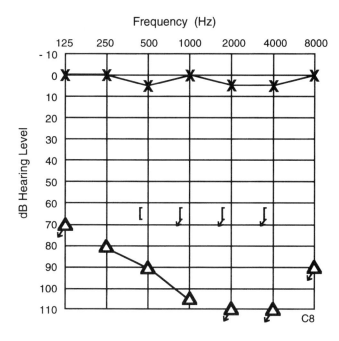

MIDDLE EAR MUSCLE REFLEXES

((⸰ ☺	Stimulus Right				☺ ⸰))	Stimulus Left			
	500	1k	2k	4k		500	1k	2k	4k
Contra	110	110	Ab	Ab	Contra	90	85	90	95
Ipsi	Ab	110	Ab	Ab	Ipsi	85	85	85	90

SPEECH AUDIOMETRY

Test Condition	Right Ear	Left Ear
Speech Awareness Threshold PB Words in Quiet	85 dB HL	96% at 40 HL

Figure 8–17. Audiometric test results for Case Study 8.

ABR RESULTS

The ABR for the left ear was obtained at 80 dB nHL at a rate of 11 clicks per second. Morphology, replicability, and absolute and interwave latencies were all normal. ABRs for the right ear were obtained for clicks presented at 80 and 90

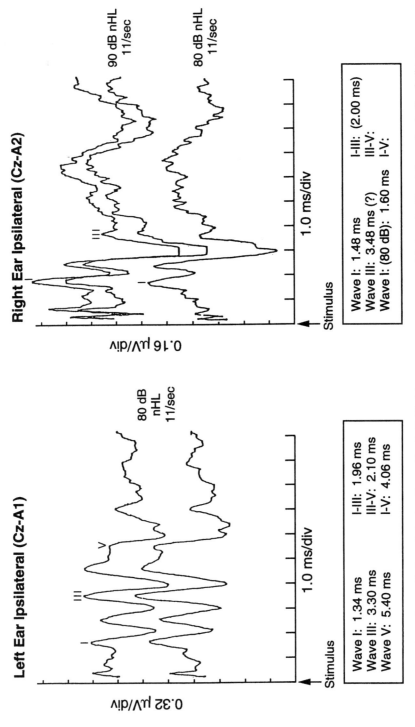

Figure 8-18. ABR results for clicks for Case Study 8. Right ear responses were obtained with white noise in the left ear.

dB nHL with and without masking in the left ear. Without masking noise in the opposite ear, a five-wave complex was obtained. However, with 66-dB SPL white noise in the left ear, only Waves I and II were present at normal latencies at 80 dB nHL, with poor synchrony beyond Wave II. When the stimulus level was increased to 90 dB nHL with 76 dB SPL noise in the left ear, a "possible" Wave V with an absolute latency at 6.8 ms was seen, which resulted in a prolonged Waves I–V interval and abnormal amplitude ratio. The ABR for the right was interpreted as markedly abnormal. The ABR results are shown in Figure 8–18.

OUTCOME

This patient had a vestibular schwannoma on the right.

COMMENT

This case demonstrates two important points related to acquisition of the ABR. First, hearing should *never* be considered too severe to attempt ABR testing. In this case, the acquisition of Waves I and II at normal latencies suggests that auditory function is normal from the external ear through the level of the cochlea and eighth nerve. The waveform after the eighth nerve response, represented by synchronous Waves I and II, is clearly abnormal. Thus, the elevated pure-tone thresholds are most likely related to the neural abnormality.

The second important point relates to the use of masking in the opposite ear when large differences in thresholds exist between the two ears. In this case, the unmasked ABR for the right ear appeared to have a Wave V, which may have reflected some components of an ABR evoked from crossover of the test stimulus to the normal-hearing ear. Applying masking to the normal ear resulted in disappearance of these later components and an ABR that properly reflected the status of the right auditory pathway.

8.9. CASE STUDY 9: ADULT WITH MENINGIOMA

HISTORY

This patient is a 66-year-old female who reported no hearing loss, with occasional dizziness and bilateral tinnitus. Case history indicated occasional headaches, nausea, and dizziness on rare occasions.

AUDIOMETRIC TEST RESULTS

Pure-tone audiometry indicated a mild low-frequency hearing loss, with other thresholds in the low-normal to mild hearing loss range bilaterally. Speech recognition in quiet was normal bilaterally. Behavioral tone decay testing was negative and the Short Increment Sensitivity Index (SISI) was 100% for the right and left ears. Audiometric test results are shown in Figure 8–19.

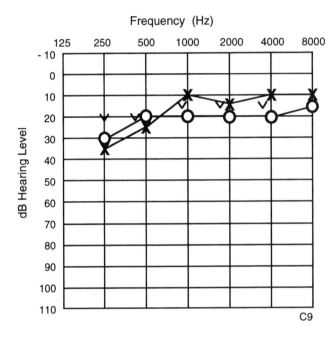

PURE TONE THRESHOLDS

MIDDLE EAR MUSCLE REFLEXES

(◖☺ Stimulus Right	500	1k	2k	4k	☺◗) Stimulus Left	500	1k	2k	4k
Contra	Ab	110	Ab	Ab	Contra	90	85	85	85
Ipsi	DNT	95	DNT	DNT	Ipsi	DNT	85	DNT	DNT

SPEECH AUDIOMETRY

Test Condition	Right Ear	Left Ear
Words in Quiet (PB Max)	96% at 55 HL	96% at 55 HL

Figure 8-19. Audiometric test results for Case Study 9.

MIDDLE EAR TEST RESULTS

Middle ear testing showed tympanograms consistent with normal middle ear function. MEMRs were normal for the left ear and elevated and absent both ipsilaterally and contralaterally when stimulating the right ear.

Although some measures were consistent with a sensory (cochlear) site, middle ear test results were suspicious, based on the elevated and absent MEMRs for the right ear. The patient was referred for ABR testing to further define the nature of the hearing problem.

ABR RESULTS

The ABR evaluation indicated normal absolute and interwave latencies for the left ear for stimuli presented at 85 dB nHL and presentation rates of 7.7, 27.7, and 57.7 stimuli per second. Best responses were obtained at 7.7 clicks per second. Responses for the right ear deviated markedly from those for the left ear and showed the presence of only Wave I at a normal latency. These results, shown in Figure 8–20, were consistent with a retrocochlear lesion on the right.

OTHER TESTS

CT scan was positive for a space-occupying lesion on the right.

OUTCOME

Surgery confirmed the presence of a large (lemon-sized) meningioma on the right side.

COMMENT

A characteristic of meningiomas is that they can grow to a large size with little effect on hearing sensitivity.

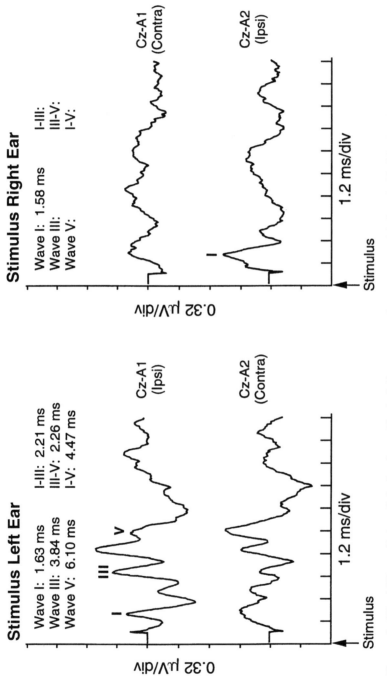

Figure 8–20. ABR results for clicks for Case Study 9. Responses shown were obtained with 85-dB nHL clicks presented at a rate of 7.7 clicks per second.

8.10. CASE STUDY 10: ADULT WITH BRAINSTEM GLIOMAS

HISTORY

This 23-year-old patient reported some balance problems and no complaint regarding hearing.

AUDIOMETRIC TEST RESULTS

Pure-tone audiometry indicated normal pure-tone thresholds for the right and left ears. Word recognition in the right ear was 88% at 40 dB HL and 92% at 90 dB HL. Word recognition in the left ear was 96% at 45 dB HL and 88% at 90 dB HL. Audiometric test results are shown in Figure 8–21.

MIDDLE EAR TEST RESULTS

Middle ear testing indicated normal tympanograms and normal ipsilateral MEMR thresholds bilaterally. However, contralateral MEMRs were absent for stimulation of both the right and left ears.

ABR RESULTS

ABRs were obtained for each ear with 80-dB nHL clicks presented at a rate of 11 stimuli per second. Results showed synchronous, replicable Waves I, II, and III that were present at normal absolute latencies. Activity following Wave III was less synchronous, with a possible low-amplitude Wave V in the right ear and no clear response after Wave III in the left ear. This ABR was interpreted as abnormal for both ears based on poor synchrony after Wave III. The ABR results are shown in Figure 8–22.

OUTCOME

This patient had multiple small lesions, identified as gliomas, in the fourth ventricle of the brainstem.

COMMENT

This patient demonstrates the importance of obtaining contralateral as well as ipsilateral MEMR responses. Had only ipsilateral reflexes been evaluated, the abnormality would have been missed. The audiological profile of normal pure-tone thresholds, normal word recognition, and normal ipsilateral and absent contralateral MEMRs is consistent with a disorder central to the eighth nerve and cochlear nuclei. This case also shows good agreement between the ABR results and MEMR pattern. Brainstem nuclei associated with crossed stapedial reflexes (e.g., the superior olivary complex) also are associated with generators of ABR components after Waves I and II.

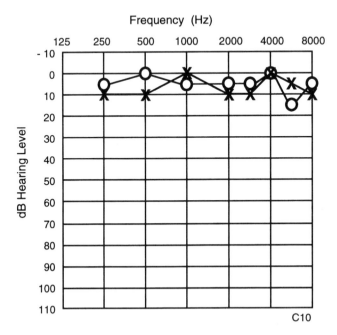

PURE TONE THRESHOLDS

MIDDLE EAR MUSCLE REFLEXES

((☺ Stimulus Right					☺)) Stimulus Left			
	500	1k	2k	4k		500	1k	2k	4k
Contra	Ab	Ab	Ab	Ab	Contra	Ab	Ab	Ab	Ab
Ipsi	80	80	85	90	Ipsi	70	80	85	90

SPEECH AUDIOMETRY

Test Condition	Right Ear	Left Ear
Words in Quiet (PB Max)	88% at 40 HL	96% at 45 HL
Words at High Intensity	92% at 90 HL	88% at 90 HL

Figure 8–21. Audiometric test results for Case Study 10.

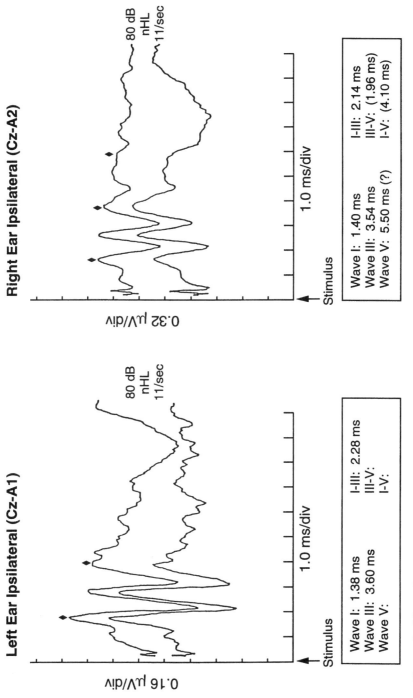

Figure 8–22. ABR results for clicks for Case Study 10.

8.11. CASE STUDY 11: INFANT WITH NORMAL HEARING

HISTORY

This infant is a 2-month-old female who was referred for evaluation because, according to family members, she did not seem to respond to or search for voices. Birth was normal, and no physical abnormalities were evident.

AUDIOMETRIC TEST RESULTS

Pure-tone audiometry was not performed due to the age of the patient.

MIDDLE EAR TEST RESULTS

Tympanograms indicated normal middle ear function, and ipsilateral and contra-lateral MEMRs were normal for both ears.

ABR RESULTS

Maximum length sequence (MLS) ABRs for air-conducted clicks were obtained first (see Figure 8–23). Standard ABR testing was completed using clicks and toneburst stimuli presented at 27.7 stimuli per second via insert earphones. Absolute and interwave latencies were prolonged for each ear at 75 dB nHL relative to adult normative values, but were within the range normally expected for infants. The latency-intensity functions for clicks and 500-Hz tonebursts indicated responses at intensities consistent with normal hearing sensitivity for the right and left ears. MLS and standard ABRs showed good agreement. Standard ABR test results for air-conducted clicks and the latency-intensity function are shown in Figures 8–24 and 8–25, respectively. ABRs obtained with 500-Hz tonebursts are shown in Figure 8–26.

OUTCOME

Test results are consistent with normal hearing sensitivity for the low- and high-frequency ranges for the right and left ears. Wave V latencies for clicks were within the normal range for infants as shown on the infant latency-intensity function. A central hearing loss cannot be ruled out based on ABR testing.

COMMENT

By obtaining responses to both clicks and low-frequency tonebursts, we were able to report information concerning hearing sensitivity for both high- and low-frequency regions of the cochlea for each ear individually. Because response thresholds for both stimuli were normal, bone conduction ABR testing was not necessary.

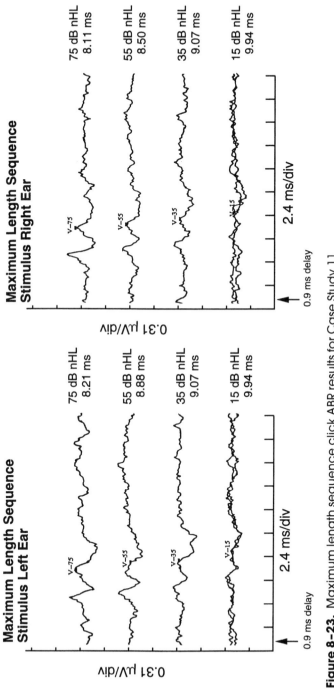

Figure 8–23. Maximum length sequence click ABR results for Case Study 11.

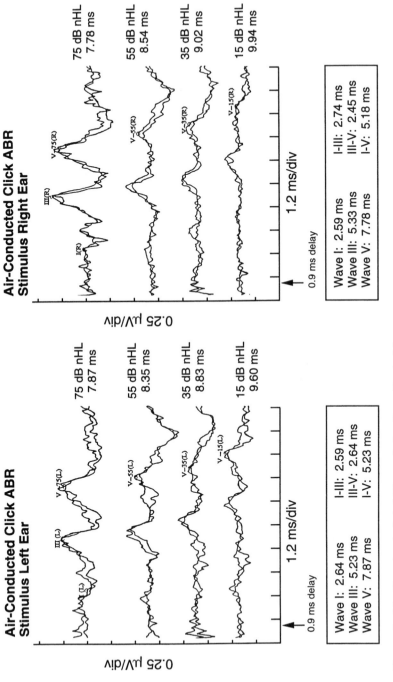

Figure 8–24. Standard click ABR results for Case Study 11.

LATENCY-INTENSITY FUNCTION FOR INFANTS

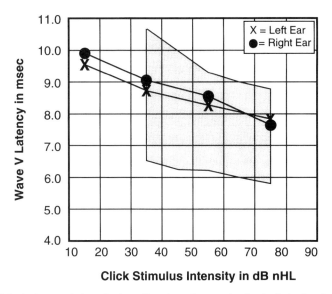

Figure 8–25. Latency-intensity function for air-conducted clicks for Case Study 11.

We often obtain latency-intensity functions using the MLS paradigm prior to standard ABR testing. This is done in case the infant becomes restless and further testing cannot be completed. With an MLS response obtained using binaural asynchronous stimuli, sensitivity for each ear to click stimuli is quickly completed and, in our experience, is consistent with standard ABR test results in threshold estimation.

8.12. CASE STUDY 12: CHILD WITH A BILATERAL CONDUCTIVE HEARING LOSS

HISTORY

This patient is a 4-year-old female who presented for testing with the following medical history: congenital heart disease that required open-heart surgery at age 1 month, delayed developmental milestones including not talking, and chronic ear infections. Previous testing by ABR at age 2 years showed a moderate conductive hearing loss that was consistent with Type B tympanograms obtained at that time. The patient has a noticeably wide inner canthus space and low-set ears.

AUDIOMETRIC AND MIDDLE EAR TEST RESULTS

This patient was referred from another clinic specifically for ABR testing. Reliable pure-tone responses could not be obtained and middle ear tests obtained from that clinic continued to be consistent with bilateral middle ear problems.

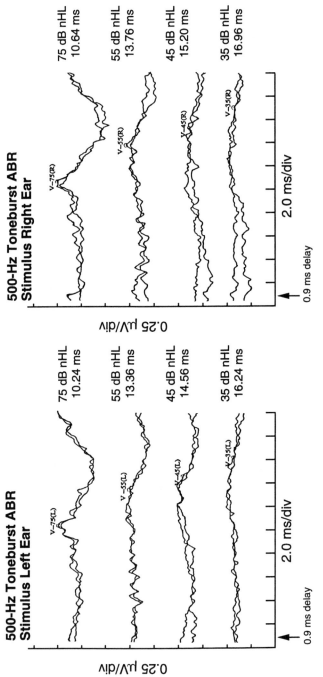

Figure 8–26. 500-Hz toneburst ABR results for Case Study 11.

ABR RESULTS

Testing was completed with the patient sedated. Air-conducted click stimuli presented via insert earphones at 27.7 clicks per second resulted in responses at intensities of 55 dB nHL and higher for the right and left ears. Interwave latencies for clicks at 75 dB nHL were normal for both ears. Responses to 500-Hz tonebursts were obtained for each ear at 75 dB nHL and above. Unmasked bone conduction responses were present at 10 dB nHL. The patient woke up before masked bone-conduction testing could be completed and only one masked response was obtained at 30 dB nHL from the left ear. ABR test results for air-conducted clicks, 500-Hz tonebursts, and bone-conducted clicks are shown in Figures 8–27, 8–28, and 8–29, respectively. Wave V latencies for air- and bone-conducted clicks are plotted on the latency-intensity function in Figure 8–30.

OUTCOME

ABR results are consistent with a moderate hearing loss in the low and high frequencies bilaterally. Unmasked bone-conduction ABR results suggest a conductive loss in at least one ear.

COMMENT

ABR testing indicated the presence of a significant hearing loss bilaterally. While masked bone conduction could not be completed, bone-conduction ABR testing was consistent with the presence of a conductive loss in at least one ear. Results of tympanometry and the medical physical examination suggested bilateral conductive involvement. Results were consistent with the ABR obtained 2 years earlier, suggesting a long-standing hearing loss that has not been successfully resolved with medical treatment and could have significant impact on development of speech and language. Although the ABR cannot rule out the possibility of a central hearing loss contributing to the patient's speech and language problems, recommendation was made that amplification be obtained as soon as possible to facilitate speech and language development.

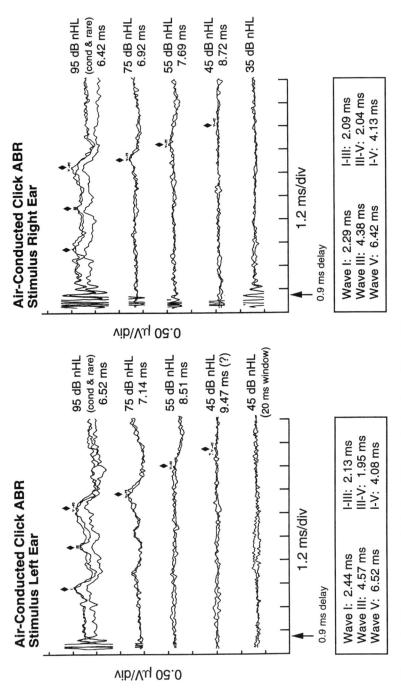

Figure 8–27. Air-conducted click ABR results for Case Study 12.

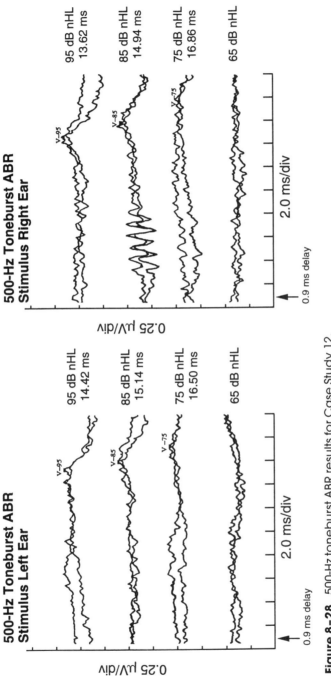

Figure 8–28. 500-Hz toneburst ABR results for Case Study 12.

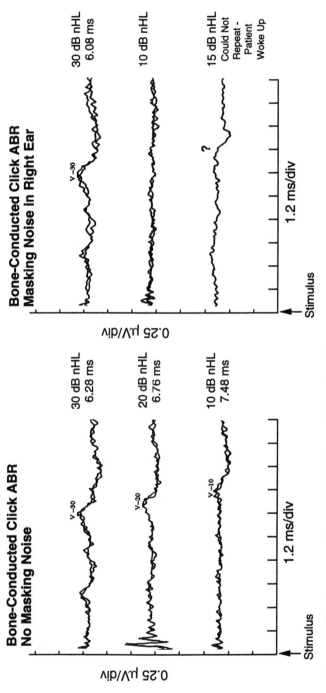

Figure 8–29. Bone-conducted click ABR results for Case Study 12.

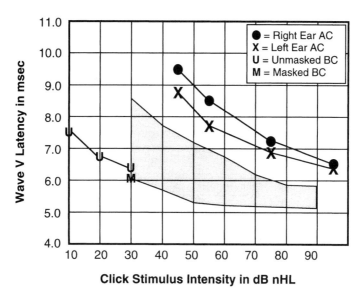

Figure 8-30. Latency-intensity function for air- and bone-conducted clicks for Case Study 12.

8.13. CASE STUDY 13: CHILD WITH UNILATERAL ATRESIA

HISTORY

This patient is a 3-year-old female who presented with a left-ear microtia and atresia. Her parents were interested in investigating reconstructive surgery; therefore quantification of sensory function in the left ear was necessary.

AUDIOMETRIC TEST RESULTS

Pure-tone audiometric results suggested normal or near normal hearing for the right ear and a large conductive loss in the left ear with normal bone conduction sensitivity. Behavioral testing with this child was difficult due to a very short attention span and inconsistent responses. Inconsistency of responses increased when masking was introduced, making cochlear sensitivity difficult to document in the left ear. The audiometric results were a composite of several test sessions. Because of questionable reliability, ABR testing was recommended. Audiometric test results are shown in Figure 8–31.

MIDDLE EAR TEST RESULTS

The tympanograms for the right ear showed −150 mm pressure, and ipsilateral MEMRs were absent for the right ear. Testing could not be completed for the left ear due to absence of an external auditory meatus.

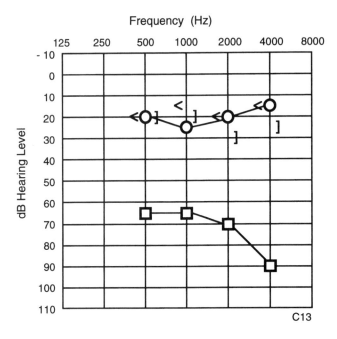

Figure 8-31. Audiometric test results for Case Study 13.

ABR RESULTS

Air-conduction click and 500-Hz toneburst results were consistent with normal hearing sensitivity for the right ear and a moderate to moderately severe hearing loss for the left ear. The right ear was masked while stimulating the left ear. Clicks were presented via bone conduction with broadband masking noise in the right ear to investigate left cochlear function. Responses were obtained at levels consistent with normal bone-conduction sensitivity in the left ear when bone-conducted clicks were presented at the forehead and the right ear was masked. The ABR results for air- and bone-conducted clicks are shown in Figures 8–32 and 8–33, respectively. Air- and bone-conducted click Wave V latencies are plotted on the latency-intensity function in Figure 8–34.

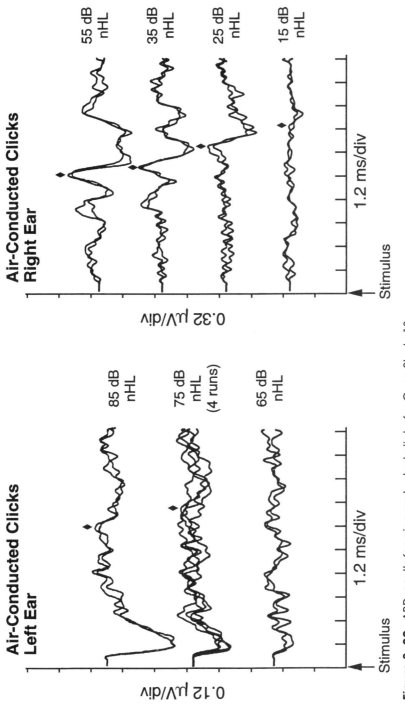

Figure 8–32. ABR results for air-conducted clicks for Case Study 13.

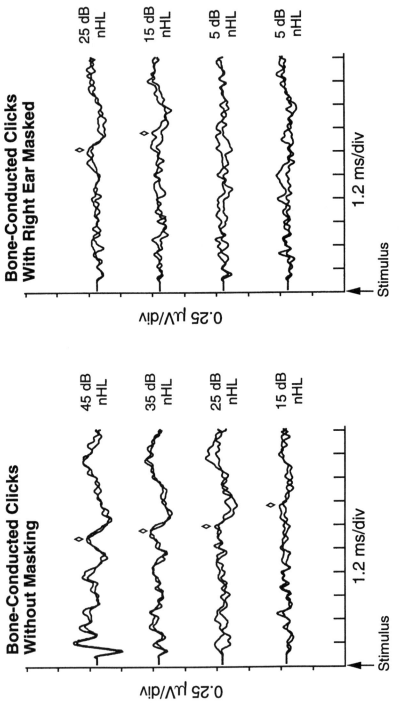

Figure 8–33. ABR results for bone-conducted clicks for Case Study 13.

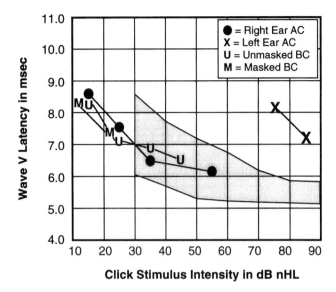

Figure 8-34. Latency-intensity function for air- and bone-conducted clicks for Case Study 13.

INTERPRETATION

ABR results were consistent with normal hearing sensitivity in the right ear and a moderately severe conductive hearing loss in the left ear.

COMMENT

In this patient, ABR testing was consistent with the results of behavioral testing and thus served as an objective and reliable cross-check of pure-tone and speech audiometry. The family was referred for further investigation of reconstructive surgery that would attempt to open or construct an external auditory canal and middle ear.

8.14. CASE STUDY 14: CHILD WITH A MODERATE SENSORY HEARING LOSS

HISTORY

This patient is a 2-year-old female whose older brother was recently diagnosed with a moderate sensorineural hearing loss.

AUDIOMETRIC TEST RESULTS

Previous audiological testing on the patient failed to obtain reliable behavioral responses to stimuli presented in the sound field. Otoacoustic emissions were absent for the right and left ears.

MIDDLE EAR TEST RESULTS

Tympanograms were normal bilaterally. Ipsilateral and contralateral MEMRs were absent for both ears.

ABR RESULTS

Air-conducted click stimuli presented at 27.7 clicks per second resulted in responses at 65 dB nHL and above for the right ear and 85 dB nHL and above for the left ear. Responses to 500-Hz tonebursts were obtained at 75 dB nHL and higher for the right ear and 95 dB nHL and higher for the left ear. Unmasked bone-conduction responses were obtained at 50 dB nHL. The ABR results for air-conducted clicks, 500-Hz tonebursts, and bone-conducted clicks are shown in Figures 8–35, 8–36, and 8–37, respectively. Response thresholds for all stimuli are summarized in Figure 8–37.

OUTCOME

The ABR results were consistent with a moderate to moderately severe hearing loss in the right ear and a moderately severe to severe hearing loss in the left ear. Following the ABR, the patient was fitted with binaural ear-level hearing aids. Subsequent behavioral pure-tone testing from ages 3 to 5 years confirmed a bilateral moderately severe sensory hearing loss (see Figure 8–38). Thresholds were 5 to 15 dB poorer in the left ear than the right ear. Aided sensitivity is in the low-normal to mild hearing loss range.

COMMENT

Obtaining objective, physiological measures of auditory sensitivity provided the information necessary to begin a management program and hopefully avoid further delays in speech and language development. Confirmation of results with behavioral testing was obtained when the child was old enough to provide reliable responses. Behavioral responses obtained at ages 3 and 5 years were consistent with the results of the ABR obtained at age 2 years.

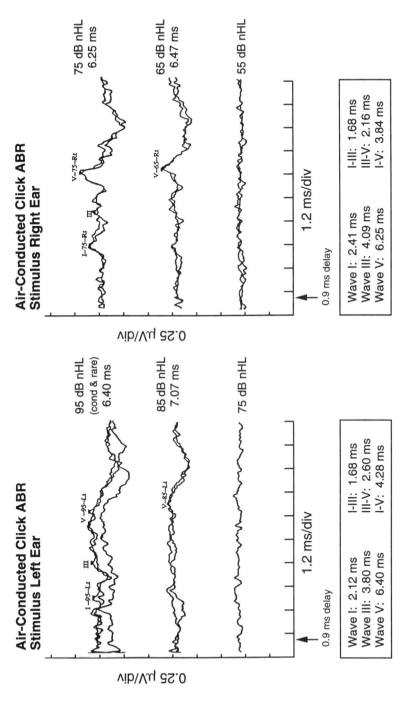

Figure 8–35. Air-conducted click ABR results for Case Study 14.

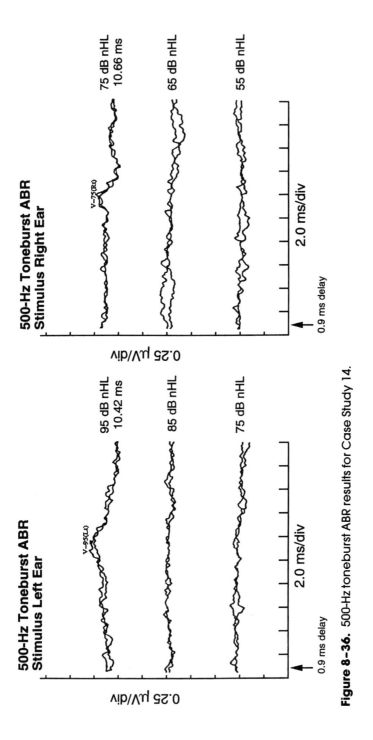

Figure 8–36. 500-Hz toneburst ABR results for Case Study 14.

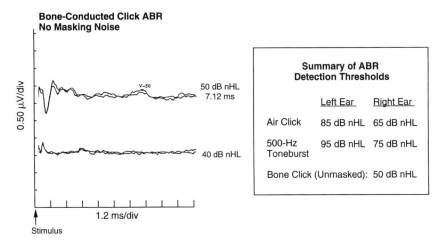

Bone-Conducted Click ABR
No Masking Noise

Summary of ABR Detection Thresholds		
	Left Ear	Right Ear
Air Click	85 dB nHL	65 dB nHL
500-Hz Toneburst	95 dB nHL	75 dB nHL
Bone Click (Unmasked):	50 dB nHL	

Figure 8–37. Bone-conducted click ABR results for Case Study 14 and summary of ABR detection thresholds.

PURE TONE THRESHOLDS

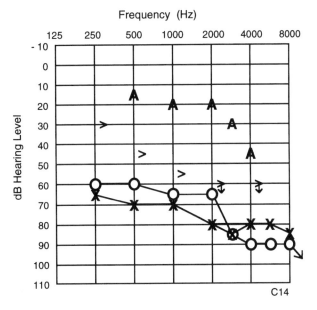

A = Aided Sound Field Thresholds for Narrow-Band Noise

SPEECH AUDIOMETRY

Test Condition	Right Ear	Left Ear
Speech Threshold (Picture Spondees)	55 dB HL	65 dB HL

Figure 8–38. Audiometric test results obtained at age 5 for Case Study 14.

8.15. CASE STUDY 15: CHILD WITH A UNILATERAL SENSORY HEARING LOSS

HISTORY

This patient is a 7-month-old female with a history of spinal meningitis.

AUDIOMETRIC TEST RESULTS

Pure-tone audiometry could not be completed. Otoacoustic emissions were present in the right ear and absent in the left ear. Transient evoked otoacoustic emissions are shown in Figure 8–39. Middle ear testing indicated a normal tympanogram for the right ear and negative middle ear pressure for the left ear. Ipsilateral MEMRs, screened at 95 dB HL, were present in the right ear and absent in the left ear.

ABR RESULTS

Maximum length sequence (MLS) ABRs showed no response in the left ear and responses at 25 dB nHL in the right ear (see Figure 8–40). With the standard ABR, responses to air-conducted clicks were obtained at 15 dB nHL in the right ear; no response was obtained at 102 dB nHL for the left ear. Testing with 500-Hz tonebursts yielded responses at 35 dB nHL in the right ear and no response at 95 dB nHL in the left ear. An unmasked response to bone-conducted clicks was obtained at 15 dB nHL. Bone-conduction testing with clicks at 50 dB nHL in the left ear and 75-dB HL masking noise in the right ear resulted in no response. The standard ABR results for air-conducted clicks, 500-Hz tonebursts, and bone-conducted clicks are shown in Figures 8–41, 8–42, and 8–43, respectively.

OUTCOME

Test results were consistent with hearing sensitivity adequate for speech development in the right ear and a severe to profound sensorineural hearing loss in the left ear. Follow-up testing in 6 to 12 months was recommended.

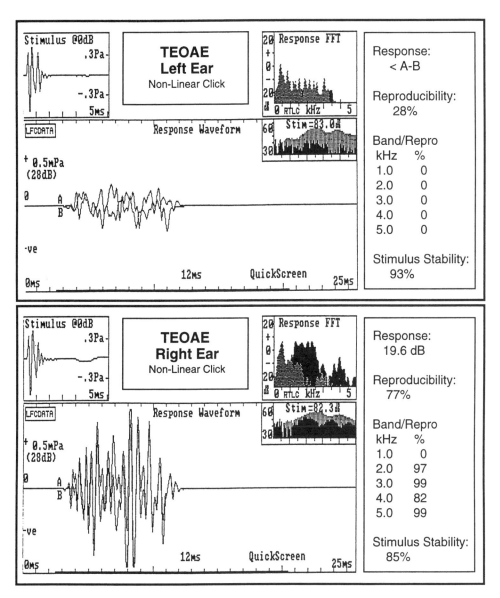

Figure 8–39. Otoacoustic emission test results for Case Study 15.

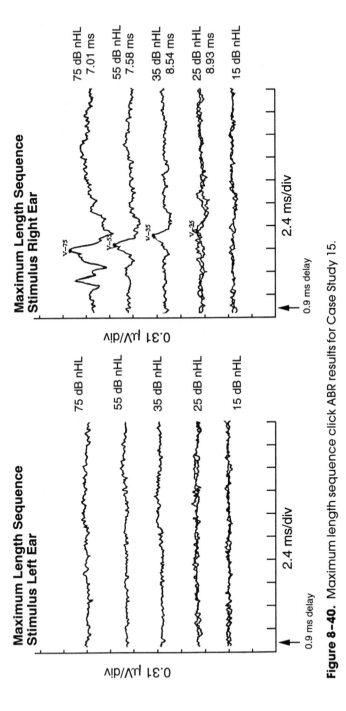

Figure 8-40. Maximum length sequence click ABR results for Case Study 15.

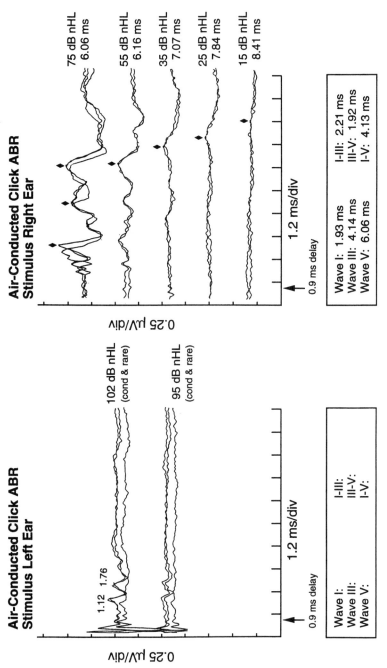

Figure 8–41. Standard air-conducted click ABR results for Case Study 15.

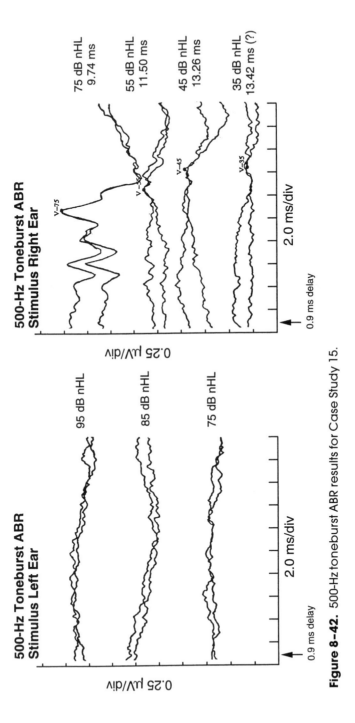

Figure 8–42. 500-Hz toneburst ABR results for Case Study 15.

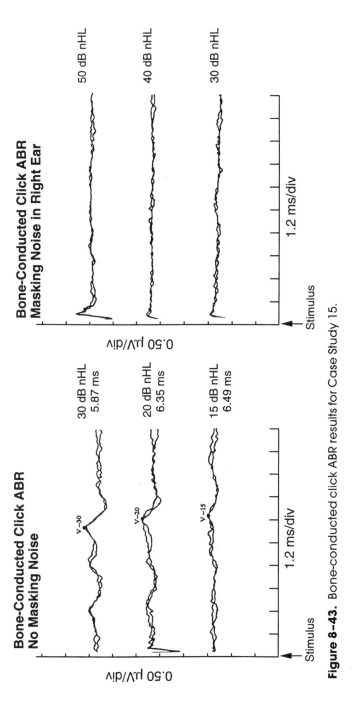

Figure 8–43. Bone-conducted click ABR results for Case Study 15.

8.16. CASE STUDY 16: ADULT WITH AN AUDITORY NEUROPATHY

HISTORY

This patient was first evaluated at age 13 years, upon failure of a school hearing test. He has been followed for the past 7 years, during which time he subsequently was diagnosed with Charcot-Marie-Tooth disease. Additional information regarding test findings for this patient can be found in articles by Berlin et al. (1993, 1994).

AUDIOMETRIC TEST RESULTS

Pure-tone audiometry at age 13 years indicated a mild to moderate high-frequency sensorineural hearing loss, which gradually decreased to a moderate to severe hearing loss over the course of several years. Word recognition has progressively decreased to poor ability to understand single words or connected speech without visual cues. Even when words could be recognized in quiet, the patient was unable to understand words or sentences presented with competing messages or noise. No masking level differences are present. Audiometric test results are shown in Figure 8–44. Robust transient evoked and distortion product otoacoustic emissions have been obtained bilaterally on all test dates (see Figure 8–45). There also is no efferent suppression of transient evoked otoacoustic emissions.

MIDDLE EAR TEST RESULTS

Tympanograms have been normal bilaterally on all tests and no ipsilateral or contralateral MEMRs have been recorded, even on earlier tests when pure-tone thresholds were normal.

AUDITORY EVOKED POTENTIAL RESULTS

No synchronous responses to ABR testing with air-conducted clicks or tone-bursts have been recorded for either ear. Cochlear responses were observed that invert with reversal of stimulus polarity (see Figure 8–46). Middle latency responses also are absent, although late responses (N1–P2 cortical potentials) are present.

OTHER TEST RESULTS

Somatosensory testing indicated reduced nerve conduction velocities, consistent with peripheral motor neuropathy characteristic of Charcot-Marie-Tooth disease.

OUTCOME

The audiological profile including the absent ABRs and present cochlear micro-phonic responses is consistent with an auditory neuropathy. An FM (frequency

PURE TONE THRESHOLDS

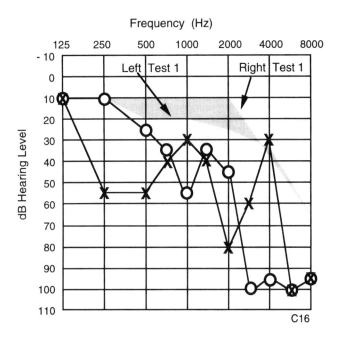

MIDDLE EAR MUSCLE REFLEXES

((· 😊	Stimulus	Right			😊 ·))	Stimulus	Left		
	500	1k	2k	4k		500	1k	2k	4k
Contra	Ab	Ab	Ab	Ab	Contra	Ab	Ab	Ab	Ab
Ipsi	Ab	Ab	Ab	Ab	Ipsi	Ab	Ab	Ab	Ab

SPEECH AUDIOMETRY

Test Condition	Right Ear	Left Ear
Words in Quiet (PB Max)	84% at 50 HL	48% at 80 HL
Words in Noise (PB Max)	0% at 50 HL	0% at 80 HL

Figure 8-44. Audiometric test results for Case Study 16.

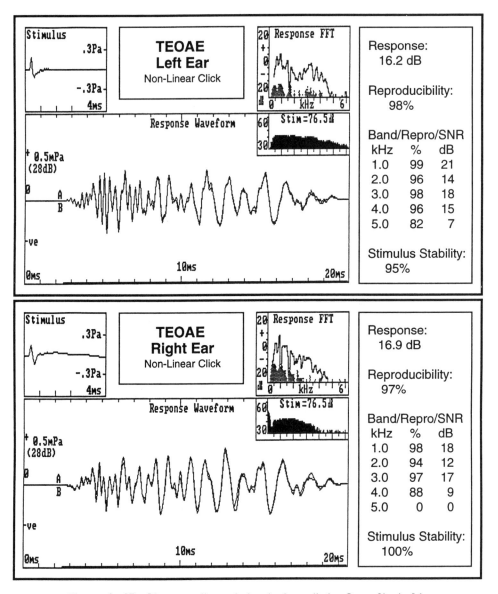

Figure 8-45. Otoacoustic emission test results for Case Study 16.

modulation) system was tried with little benefit. The patient depends primarily on lipreading and other visual cues for communication.

COMMENT

An absent ABR in the presence of normal otoacoustic emissions is the classic indicator of an auditory neuropathy. The characteristics of auditory neuropathy are described in Chapter 5 (see Section 5.4.3.1).

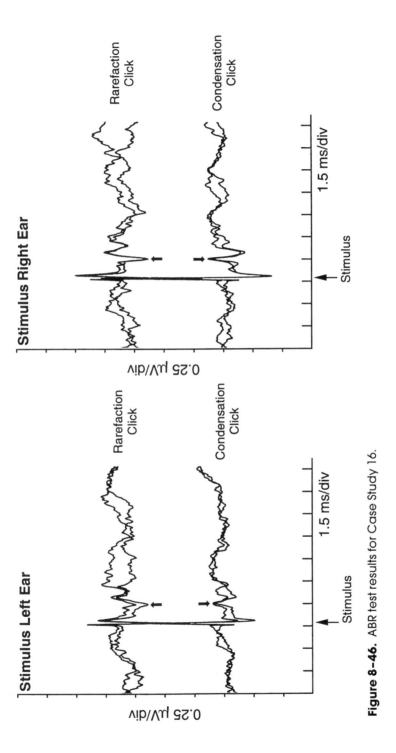

Figure 8–46. ABR test results for Case Study 16.

8.17. CASE STUDY 17: INFANT WITH AN AUDITORY NEUROPATHY

HISTORY

This patient is one of a pair of twins who were born at 34 weeks' gestation by cesarean section due to fetal distress. Birthweight was 3 lbs 8.7 oz. The patient had a stormy birth and early history including anemia, oxygen therapy, three transfusions, phototherapy for high bilirubin levels, and a Grade IV intraventricular hemorrhage. The patient also was the donor in a twin-to-twin transfusion. Additional information regarding history and test findings for this patient can be found in an article by Berlin et al. (1998).

OTOACOUSTIC EMISSIONS

Transient evoked otoacoustic emissions, obtained at age 5½ months, were present bilaterally (see Figure 8–47).

ABR RESULTS

Due to a number of high-risk indicators, initial ABR testing completed at another center on hospital discharge showed no response using alternating-polarity clicks. The infant was referred to our center to "confirm deafness and fit hearing aids."

An ABR was obtained without sedation at age 4 months. Questionable responses were obtained at 75 dB nHL for clicks, and no responses were obtained for 500-Hz tonebursts or bone-conducted clicks. Reliability of testing was questioned due to patient restlessness. Plans were made to obtain an ABR and otoacoustic emissions with sedation.

An ABR with sedation was obtained when the infant was just under 6 months of age. These results are shown in Figures 8–48 and 8–49. Responses to condensation clicks showed replicable activity over a 6- to 8-ms time period poststimulus for each ear at stimulus intensities of 75 dB nHL and above. Close examination of the responses showed expected decreases in response amplitude with decreasing stimulus intensities, but *no* increase in latency of the response peaks (see Figure 8–48). When stimulus polarity was reversed, the response inverted (see Figure 8–49). This is characteristic of a cochlear response rather than a neural response.

OUTCOME

The otoacoustic emission and ABR test results are consistent with an auditory neuropathy. The family has been encouraged to use either Cued Speech or signing if learning by auditory means does not seem to facilitate speech and language development. The patient and his twin do not use hearing aids, but do use

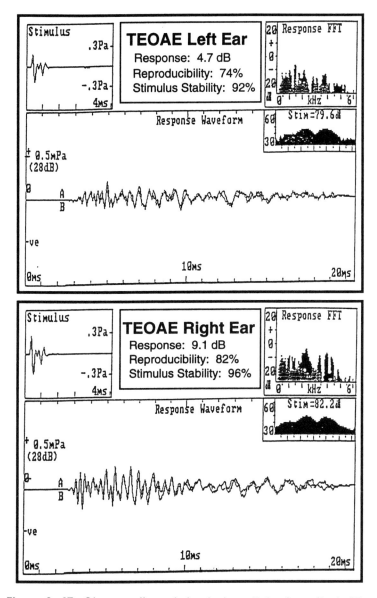

Figure 8-47. Otoacoustic emission test results for Case Study 17.

assistive listening devices and receive speech/language intervention to facilitate development. Some signs are used to support language comprehension, and the parents report some responses to speech.

COMMENT

A somewhat surprising number of infants and young children have been identified with an auditory neuropathy. Correct identification, as discussed in Chapter

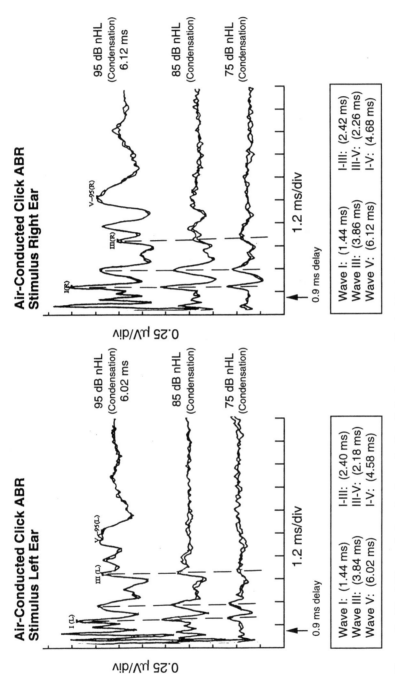

Figure 8–48. ABR results for single-polarity clicks for Case Study 17. Note that markings of Waves I, III, and V latencies on waveforms are not true neural responses (see Figure 8–49).

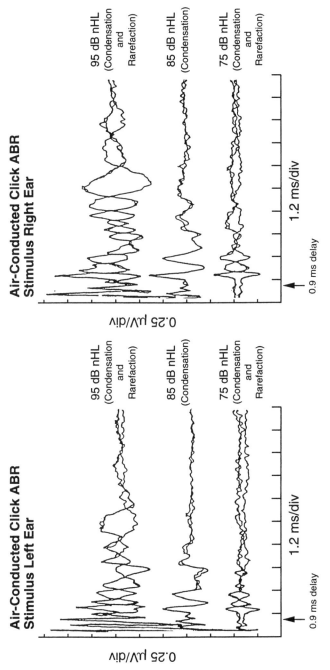

Figure 8–49. Click ABR results with polarity reversed for Case Study 17.

7 (Section 7.6), depends on comparison of ABRs obtained using condensation clicks to those obtained using rarefaction clicks in order to distinguish cochlear from neural components. The combination of no neural response on the ABR coupled with normal otoacoustic emissions and/or the presence of the cochlear microphonic is a definitive finding. Management issues for this population, as discussed in Chapter 7, present particular challenges to the clinician.

8.18. CASE STUDY 18: COLLAPSED EAR CANAL THAT MIMICS A RETROCOCHLEAR LESION

HISTORY

This case describes test results for an 8-year-old male who was recruited to participate in a research study as a member of a group of supposedly normal children. Birth and developmental history were normal, and there was no suspicion of any auditory problem.

AUDIOMETRIC TEST RESULTS

Pure-tone thresholds were within normal limits for both ears, although high-frequency thresholds were slightly higher in the left than in the right ear. Speech reception thresholds were normal bilaterally and speech recognition for monosyllables was 96% at 45 and 50 dB HL for the right and left ears, respectively. Audiometric test results are shown in Figure 8–50.

MIDDLE EAR TEST RESULTS

Tympanograms were consistent with normal middle ear function, and MEMRs were in the normal to slightly above normal range. The contralateral reflex threshold at 4000 Hz in the left ear was elevated. Reflex decay was negative at 1000 Hz in each ear.

ABR RESULTS

ABR results indicated normal absolute and interwave latencies for the right ear. The morphology for the left ear response was quite different from the right ear and showed prolonged Waves III and V latencies. Although Waves III and V could be identified in the left ear, Wave I was difficult to discern. A second test was performed using a different evoked potential system, and results confirmed the findings of the first ABR with a significantly prolonged Wave V for the left ear (see Figure 8–51). Both of these ABR systems were configured with aural dome earphones. A third test was then performed with a third evoked potential system that was configured with lightweight nonoccluding earphones (Koss HV/X). Normal ABRs were obtained for the right and left ears.

PURE TONE THRESHOLDS

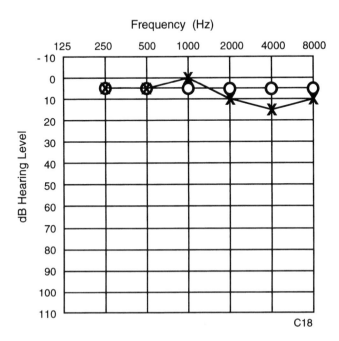

MIDDLE EAR MUSCLE REFLEXES

((☺) Stimulus Right	500	1k	2k	4k	(☺)) Stimulus Left	500	1k	2k	4k
Contra	90	90	95	90	Contra	90	100	95	115
Ipsi	100	95	90	DNT	Ipsi	100	95	90	DNT

SPEECH AUDIOMETRY

Test Condition	Right Ear	Left Ear
Words in Quiet (PB Max)	96% at 45 HL	96% at 50 HL

Figure 8–50. Audiometric test results for Case Study 18.

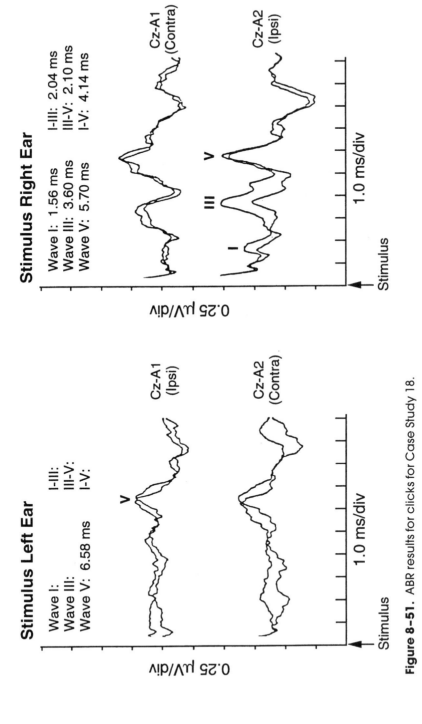

Figure 8–51. ABR results for clicks for Case Study 18.

OUTCOME

Normal ABR.

COMMENT

This case emphasizes the need to eliminate sources of technical error in acquiring and interpreting test results. The aural dome earphones used in tests 1 and 2 resulted in collapse of the left ear canal and introduction of a "conductive" hearing loss with a Wave I too small to read. When smaller, lighter weight earphones were used, normal responses were obtained for both ears. Insert phones are ideal for preventing this kind of error, as well as reducing the need for masking. Other clues, in retrospect, to the collapsed ear canal are the poorer high frequency pure-tone and contralateral MEMR thresholds in the left ear.

8.19. CASE STUDY 19: POSTAURICULAR MUSCLE ARTIFACT

HISTORY

This patient is a 49-year-old female who reported a hearing loss with better hearing in her left ear, tinnitus in the right ear, and difficulty hearing in groups and noisy situations. She further reported dizzy spells once or twice per week, sometimes accompanied by nausea. Results of a glycerin test were negative.

AUDIOMETRIC TEST RESULTS

Pure-tone audiometry indicated a moderate hearing loss rising to a mild loss in the higher frequencies in the right ear and a mild hearing loss in the left ear. Speech thresholds were consistent with pure-tone results, and speech recognition for monosyllables in quiet was reduced for the right (76% at 80 dB HL) and left (88% at 55 dB HL) ears. Word recognition in the right ear was 80% at 90 dB HL and 64% at 100 dB HL. Audiometric test results are shown in Figure 8–52.

MIDDLE EAR TEST RESULTS

Middle ear testing showed normal tympanograms and contralateral MEMRs bilaterally.

ABR RESULTS

Initially, a large number of sweeps were rejected, despite observation of a relaxed, quiet patient. A high amplitude peak was noted in the 8- to 12-ms time range in the right contralateral response, which prevented acquisition of a sufficient number of averages. When the artifact rejection system was disabled, recording could be completed. A second set of responses was obtained using a 7-ms time window

PURE TONE THRESHOLDS

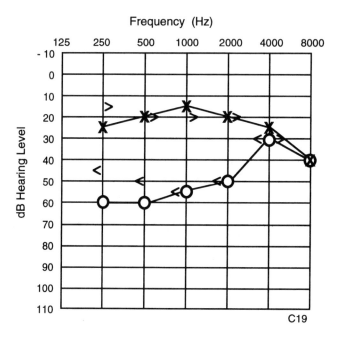

C19

MIDDLE EAR MUSCLE REFLEXES

((☺ Stimulus Right	500	1k	2k	4k	☺)) Stimulus Left	500	1k	2k	4k
Contra	80	85	85	80	Contra	85	90	90	90
Ipsi	DNT	DNT	DNT	DNT	Ipsi	DNT	DNT	DNT	DNT

SPEECH AUDIOMETRY

Test Condition	Right Ear	Left Ear
Words in Quiet (PB Max)	76% at 80 HL	88% at 55 HL

Figure 8–52. Audiometric test results for Case Study 19.

that did not include the postauricular muscle (PAM) artifact observed between 8 and 12 ms and allowed utilization of the artifact rejection system. The ABR results obtained for 12-ms and 7-ms time windows are shown in Figures 8–53 and 8–54, respectively.

OUTCOME

Understanding the stimulus, recording, and subject characteristics of the ABR is helpful in troubleshooting during recording. Recognizing possible sources of interference in recordings (such as electrical or myogenic artifact) allows appropriate measures to be taken to reduce the interference. In this case with muscle artifact, either the artifact rejection system could be disabled or the time window could be shortened. The clinician chose to shorten the time window as the first strategy. Had the response shown prolonged components, shortening the window might not have been possible. In that case, the artifact rejection system could have been disabled and, though less efficient, large amplitude sweeps could have been monitored manually.

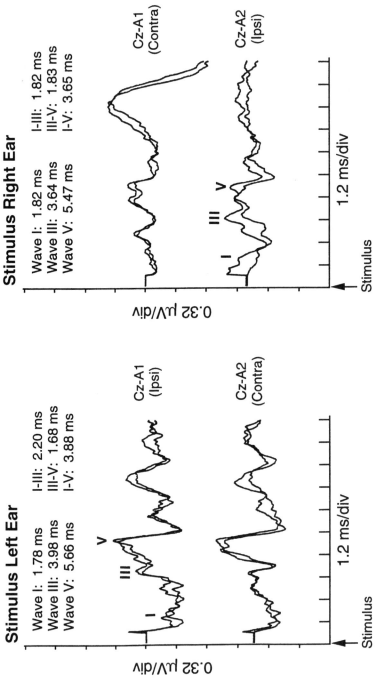

Figure 8–53. ABR results for clicks using a 12-ms time window for Case Study 19.

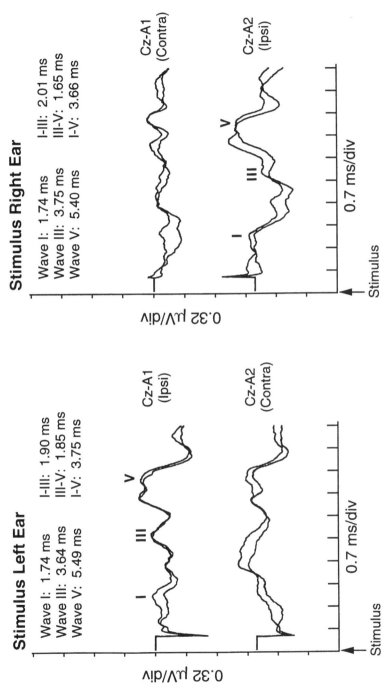

Figure 8–54. ABR results for clicks using a 7-ms time window for Case Study 19.

8.20. CASE STUDY 20: TECHNICAL ERROR IN ELECTRODE CONNECTION

HISTORY

This patient is a 25-year-old female who was recruited for collection of normative data. No history of middle ear disorders, noise exposure, or any auditory difficulties was reported.

AUDIOMETRIC TEST RESULTS

Pure-tone audiometry indicated normal hearing sensitivity bilaterally, as shown in Figure 8–55. Word recognition was normal for both ears.

MIDDLE EAR TEST RESULTS

Middle ear testing showed normal tympanograms and MEMR thresholds bilaterally.

ABR RESULTS

The initial ABR indicated an unusual morphology, and it was difficult to distinguish the usual ABR peaks (see Figure 8–56). Because of this finding, a check was made to be sure that the clicks were audible and that the electrodes were correctly connected. It was discovered that the electrodes were improperly connected with the vertex and earlobe electrodes inverted. When the electrodes were correctly connected, a normal ABR recording was obtained (Figure 8–57).

COMMENT

This case demonstrates the importance of carefully checking the stimulus and recording setup throughout testing. Whenever recordings are unusual or difficult to interpret, the first strategy should be to rule out a technical error. If the patient is awake, it is good practice to ask the patient if the stimulus is present in the proper earphone. Electrode connections should be checked both for correct routing from the patient to the electrode interface and for consistency with the electrode configuration identified in the computer setup.

PURE TONE THRESHOLDS

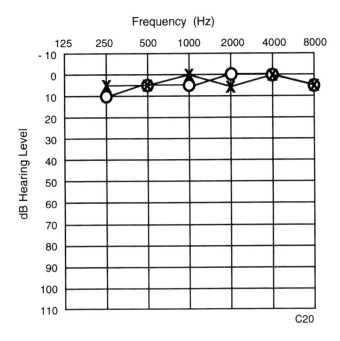

MIDDLE EAR MUSCLE REFLEXES

(◖ ☺	Stimulus Right				☺ ◗)	Stimulus Left			
	500	1k	2k	4k		500	1k	2k	4k
Contra	85	80	85	85	Contra	80	85	85	90
Ipsi	85	85	80	85	Ipsi	80	85	80	85

SPEECH AUDIOMETRY

Test Condition	Right Ear	Left Ear
Words in Quiet (PB Max)	100% at 45 HL	100% at 45 HL

Figure 8-55. Audiometric test results for Case Study 20.

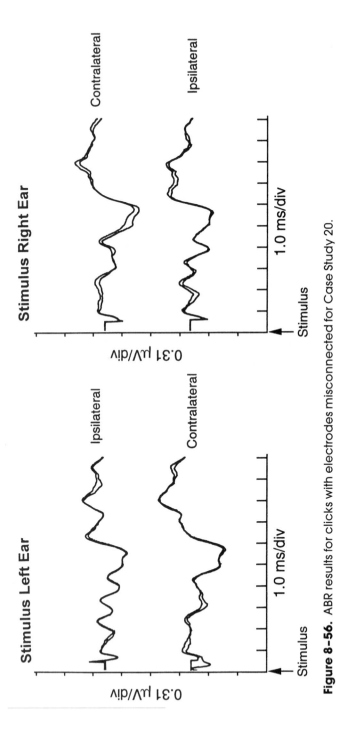

Figure 8–56. ABR results for clicks with electrodes misconnected for Case Study 20.

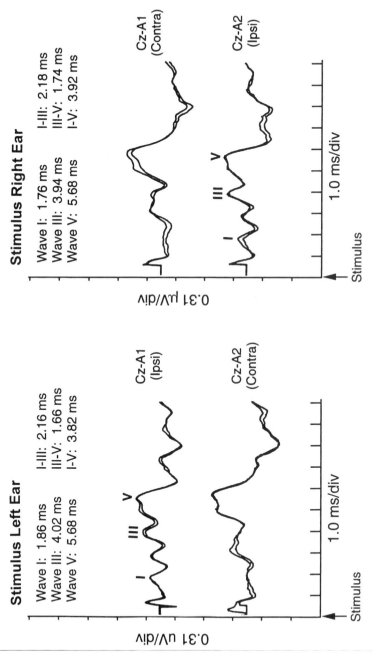

Stimulus Left Ear

Wave I: 1.86 ms   I-III: 2.16 ms
Wave III: 4.02 ms   III-V: 1.66 ms
Wave V: 5.68 ms   I-V: 3.82 ms

Cz-A1 (Ipsi)

Cz-A2 (Contra)

0.31 uV/div

1.0 ms/div

Stimulus

Stimulus Right Ear

Wave I: 1.76 ms   I-III: 2.18 ms
Wave III: 3.94 ms   III-V: 1.74 ms
Wave V: 5.68 ms   I-V: 3.92 ms

Cz-A1 (Contra)

Cz-A2 (Ipsi)

0.31 uV/div

1.0 ms/div

Stimulus

Figure 8–57. ABR results for clicks with electrodes correctly connected for Case Study 20.

Reporting ABR Test Results

Accurate and complete reports of test results are a critical part of the auditory brainstem response (ABR) evaluation. Included in this section are some examples of reports of ABR test results for children and adults with normal and abnormal findings that may serve as a basis for developing a report format. We try to limit our reports to a one-page summary of results and *always* include copies of the actual ABR waveforms with the latencies marked and summarized in a table. Most clinical ABR systems provide a format for plotting and marking waveforms and also print a table summarizing the latency (and amplitude) measures. We enclose this with our verbal report.

Remember to: 1. Include copies of the ABR waveforms.
2. Include the test parameters.
3. Include latency values and show on the waveforms where the latencies were marked.

9.1. ABR TESTING FOR ESTIMATION OF PERIPHERAL HEARING SENSITIVITY

The first three reports are samples of ABR results obtained when the primary purpose of the ABR was to obtain an estimate of hearing sensitivity. Absolute and interwave latencies are also reported as an assessment of neural integrity.

9.1.1. Sample Infant/Child Report—Consistent With Normal Peripheral Sensitivity

Report of Auditory Brainstem Response Evaluation

(Patient Name) was seen for auditory brainstem response (ABR) testing on (test date). The (infant/child) presented with the following medical history:

_____

Middle ear measures indicated normal tympanograms and ipsilateral and contralateral middle ear muscle reflexes were within normal limits. Otoacoustic emissions were consistent with normal cochlear function. These measures were completed just prior to ABR testing.

ABR testing was completed with air-conducted clicks presented to each ear through insert earphones at a rate of 27.7 per second. Testing at an intensity level of 75 dB nHL indicated absolute and interwave latencies that were within age-appropriate normative values. Responses to air-conducted clicks were obtained at decreasing intensities down to 15 dB nHL in each ear. ABRs to 500-Hz tonebursts were obtained at intensities down to 35 dB nHL for each ear. Copies of marked waveforms and a summary table of absolute and interwave latencies are enclosed.

These results are consistent with normal and/or adequate peripheral hearing sensitivity for speech development.

Note: There are occasionally children who show good ABR responses who have either central or related auditory deficits. Please call us again if this patient fails to develop speech and language as predicted.

9.1.2. Sample Infant/Child Report—Consistent With Moderate Conductive Hearing Loss

Report of Auditory Brainstem Response Evaluation

(Patient Name) was seen for auditory brainstem response (ABR) testing on (test date). The (infant/child) presented with the following medical history:

_____

Middle ear measures indicated Type B tympanograms and absent ipsilateral and contralateral middle ear muscle reflexes bilaterally. Otoacoustic emissions were not present. These measures were completed just prior to ABR testing.

ABR testing was completed with air-conducted clicks presented to each ear through insert earphones at a rate of 27.7 per second. Testing at an intensity level of 75 dB nHL indicated prolonged absolute latencies for Waves I, III, and V. Interwave latencies were within age-appropriate normative values. Responses to air-conducted clicks were obtained at decreasing intensities down to 55 dB nHL in each ear. ABRs to 500-Hz tonebursts were obtained at intensity levels down to 65 dB nHL for each ear. Responses to bone-conducted clicks presented with masking noise in the opposite ear were obtained at intensity levels of 15 dB nHL for each ear. Copies of marked waveforms and a summary table of absolute and interwave latencies are enclosed.

ABRs to air-conducted clicks and 500-Hz tonebursts are consistent with a moderate hearing loss in the low- and high-frequency ranges for the right and left ears. Normal ABRs to bone-conducted clicks suggest a bilateral conductive hearing loss.

Appropriate medical follow-up and management are recommended.

Note: There are occasionally children who show ABR responses who have either central or related auditory deficits. Please call us again if this patient fails to develop speech and language as predicted.

9.1.3. Sample Infant/Child Report—Consistent With Mild to Moderate Cochlear Hearing Loss

---

Report of Auditory Brainstem Response Evaluation

(Patient Name) was seen for auditory brainstem response (ABR) testing on (test date). The (infant/child) presented with the following medical history:

_____

Middle ear measures indicated normal tympanograms bilaterally and ipsilateral and contralateral middle ear muscle reflexes were within normal limits. Otoacoustic emissions were absent for both ears. These measures were completed just prior to ABR testing.

ABR testing was completed with air-conducted clicks presented to each ear through insert earphones at a rate of 27.7 per second. Testing at an intensity level of 75 dB nHL indicated absolute and interwave latencies that were within age-appropriate normative values. Responses to air-conducted clicks were obtained at intensities of 50 dB nHL and higher in each ear. ABRs to 500-Hz tonebursts were obtained at intensities of 45 dB nHL and higher for each ear. Responses to unmasked bone-conducted clicks were obtained at 45 dB nHL. Copies of marked waveforms and a summary table of absolute and interwave latencies are enclosed.

ABRs to air-conducted clicks and 500-Hz tonebursts are consistent with a mild to moderate hearing loss in the right and left ears that is greater in the higher frequencies. Elevated response levels for bone-conducted clicks are consistent with a bilateral cochlear hearing loss. ABR results are consistent with otoacoustic emissions and middle ear test results.

If not already done, the patient should be considered for hearing aids and auditory (re)habilitation as soon as possible.

Note: There are occasionally children who show ABR responses who have either central or related auditory deficits. Please call us again if this patient fails to develop as predicted.

9.2. ABR TESTING FOR OTONEUROLOGICAL EVALUATION

The following three reports are samples of ABR results obtained when the primary purpose of the ABR was to obtain information related to otoneurological evaluation. Absolute and interwave latencies are reported as an assessment of neural integrity. Adult patients are the usual target of use of the ABR for otoneurological evaluation. Patients with and without peripheral hearing loss are included.

9.2.1. Sample Adult Report—Normal Peripheral Hearing and Normal ABR

Report of Auditory Brainstem Response Evaluation

(Patient Name) was seen for otoneurological evaluation with the auditory brainstem response (ABR) on (test date). The patient presented with the following history and symptoms:

_____

Audiometric test results indicated normal hearing sensitivity for the right and left ears. Middle ear measures indicated normal tympanograms and ipsilateral and contralateral middle ear muscle reflexes were within normal limits. Otoacoustic emissions were consistent with normal cochlear function.

ABR testing was completed with air-conducted clicks presented to each ear through insert earphones at rates of 7.7, 27.7, and 57.7 per second and an intensity level of 75 dB nHL. Copies of marked waveforms and a summary table of absolute and interwave latencies are enclosed.

Results of ABR testing are interpreted as normal. This interpretation is based on normal absolute and interwave latencies for both ears, a normal comparison of latencies between ears, and a normal shift of Wave V latency with increased stimulus repetition rate.

9.2.2. Sample Adult Report—ABR Consisient With Bilateral Moderately Severe High-Frequency Peripheral Hearing Loss

---

Report of Auditory Brainstem Response Evaluation

(Patient Name) was seen for otoneurological evaluation with the auditory brainstem response (ABR) on (test date). The patient presented with the following history and symptoms:

_____

Audiometric test results indicated a mild hearing loss through 1500 Hz, with a moderately severe high-frequency hearing loss for the right and left ears. Middle ear measures indicated normal tympanograms and ipsilateral and contralateral middle ear muscle reflexes were elevated in the high frequencies, consistent with audiometric thresholds. Otoacoustic emissions were absent, which is consistent with cochlear hearing loss.

ABR testing was completed with air-conducted clicks presented to each ear through insert earphones at rates of 7.7, 27.7, and 57.7 per second and an intensity level of 85 dB nHL. Copies of marked waveforms and a summary table of absolute and interwave latencies are enclosed.

Results of ABR testing are interpreted as consistent with a cochlear hearing loss. This interpretation is based on prolonged absolute latencies for Waves I, III, and V with normal interwave latencies for both ears, a normal comparison of latencies between ears, and a normal shift of Wave V latency with increased stimulus repetition rate.

Recommendation is made that this patient obtain follow-up management with appropriate amplification.

9.2.3. Sample Adult Report—Abnormal ABR Consistent With Eighth Nerve/Brainstem Lesion

---

Report of Auditory Brainstem Response Evaluation

(Patient Name) was seen for otoneurological evaluation with the auditory brainstem response (ABR) on (test date). The patient presented with the following history and symptoms:

_____

Audiometric test results indicated normal hearing sensitivity for the right ear and a mild high-frequency hearing loss for the left ear. Middle ear measures indicated normal tympanograms bilaterally and ipsilateral and contralateral middle ear muscle reflexes were within normal limits for stimulation of the right ear and elevated and absent on stimulation of the left ear. Otoacoustic emissions were present in both ears.

ABR testing was completed with air-conducted clicks presented to each ear through insert earphones at rates of 7.7, 27.7, and 57.7 per second and an intensity level of 75 dB nHL. Copies of marked waveforms and a summary table of absolute and interwave latencies are enclosed.

Results of ABR testing are interpreted as normal for the right ear and abnormal for the left ear. The abnormal findings for the left ear are based on prolonged absolute latencies for Waves III and V and prolonged I-III and I-V interwave latencies.

Recommendation is made that imaging studies and medical follow-up be obtained.

ABR Laboratory Exercises and Protocol Practice

I. LABORATORY EXERCISES

1. Normal Auditory Brainstem Response
2. Effects of Stimulus Intensity
3. Effects of Stimulus Polarity
4. Effects of Presentation Rate
5. Comparison of Electrode Montages
6. Effects of Filter Settings
7. 500-Hz Toneburst ABR
8. Bone Conduction ABR
9. 40-Hz Response Using a 500-Hz Toneburst

II. PROTOCOL PRACTICE

1. Neurological Application
2. Estimation of Hearing Sensitivity in Infants
3. Estimation of Hearing Sensitivity in Older Children or Adults

III. SKILL CHECKLIST

I. LABORATORY EXERCISES

1. Normal Auditory Brainstem Response

In this exercise, a two-channel ABR will be recorded. Replication of all responses (i.e., test and retest runs) should be obtained for this and all of the following exercises. Absolute latencies, interwave latencies, and amplitude will be determined and compared to normative data.

Normal Auditory Brainstem Response

Parameter	Setup
Stimulus type	Click
Stimulus polarity	Condensation or rarefaction
Intensity	75 dB nHL
Presentation rate	27.7/second
Time base	12 ms
Filter band	100–3000 Hz
Electrode montage	C_Z–A_1, C_Z–A_2
Number of channels	2
Number of sweeps	1500 or F_{SP}

RESULTS:

		Left Ear	Right Ear
Latency:	Wave I	_____	_____
	Wave III	_____	_____
	Wave V	_____	_____
	Waves I–III	_____	_____
	Waves III–V	_____	_____
	Waves I–V	_____	_____
Amplitude:	Wave I–I'	_____	_____
	Wave V–V'	_____	_____
	Wave V/I	_____	_____

NOTES: The two replications (test and retest runs) should be compared for consistency. Waves I, III, and V should be present in a normal response from a normal-hearing subject. The absolute latencies of Waves I, III, and V should be marked on the ipsilateral responses for the right and left ears. Calculate the interwave latencies by comparing the latencies of the appropriate waves (e.g., Waves I and III for the I–III interval). To calculate the Wave V/I amplitude, determine the peak-to-peak amplitude from the peak to the following trough of Wave I and Wave V. Use the higher of the Waves IV and V amplitude for the positive amplitude value for Wave V. Then divide the peak-to-peak amplitude of Wave V by the peak-to-peak amplitude of Wave I. (See Figures 2–1, 2–2, and 2–7.)

2. Effects of Stimulus Intensity

In this exercise, ABRs will be obtained using air-conduction clicks at a series of intensities from high to low intensity. Absolute latencies, interwave latencies, and amplitude will be determined for all waves present. A Wave V latency-intensity function will be plotted.

Effects of Stimulus Intensity

Parameter	Setup
Stimulus type	Click
Stimulus polarity	Condensation
Intensity	*75, 55, 35, 15 dB nHL*
Presentation rate	27.7/second
Time base	12 ms
Filter band	100–3000 Hz
Electrode montage	C_z–A_1, C_z–A_2
Number of channels	2
Number of sweeps	1500 or F_{SP}

RESULTS:

		__ dB nHL	__ dB nHL	__ dB nHL	__ dB nHL
Intensity:					
Latency:	Wave I				
	Wave III				
	Wave V				
	Waves I–III				
	Waves III–V				
	Waves I–V				
Amplitude:	Wave I–I'				
	Wave V–V'				
	Wave V/I				

NOTES: Latency should increase and amplitude should decrease as intensity is lowered. At high intensities all components should be present. At lower intensities the earlier waves may not be present. (See Figure 2–3.)

Wave V latency-intensity function. Plot the absolute latency of Wave V for each of the intensity levels tested on the latency-intensity function. (See Figures 2–4 and A–1.)

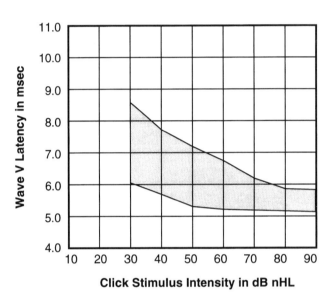

LATENCY-INTENSITY FUNCTION FOR ADULTS

(Based on +/- 3 standard deviations, young females)

Figure A-1. Adult latency-intensity function.

3. Effects of Stimulus Polarity

In this exercise, two-channel ABRs will be recorded using condensation and rarefaction click stimuli. Absolute latencies, interwave latencies, and amplitude will be determined.

Effects of Stimulus Polarity

Parameter	Setup
Stimulus type	Click
Stimulus polarity	*Condensation*
	Rarefaction
Intensity	75 dB nHL
Presentation rate	27.7/second
Time base	12 ms
Filter band	100–3000 Hz
Electrode montage	C_Z–A_1, C_Z–A_2
Number of channels	2
Number of sweeps	1500 or F_{SP}

RESULTS:

Stimulus Polarity:		Condensation	Rarefaction
Latency:	Wave I	_____	_____
	Wave III	_____	_____
	Wave V	_____	_____
	Waves I–III	_____	_____
	Waves III–V	_____	_____
	Waves I–V	_____	_____
Amplitude:	Wave I–I'	_____	_____
	Wave V–V'	_____	_____
	Wave V/I	_____	_____

NOTES: Comparison of averages obtained using condensation and rarefaction clicks may show slight differences in latency and amplitude for various components of the ABR. In many but not all subjects, rarefaction clicks result in a slightly earlier and higher amplitude Wave I whereas condensation clicks yield slightly longer latencies and higher amplitude of Wave V. If the cochlear microphonic is present (preceding Wave I), that part of the response should reverse with polarity changes. (See Figures 3–5 and 4–1.)

4. Effects of Presentation Rate

In this exercise, two-channel ABRs will be recorded using click stimuli at four different stimulus rates. Absolute latencies, interwave latencies, and amplitude will be determined.

Effects of Presentation Rate	
Parameter	**Setup**
Stimulus type	Click
Stimulus polarity	Condensation or rarefaction
Intensity	75 dB nHL
Presentation rate	*7.7, 27.7, 57.7, 77.7 per second*
Time base	12 ms
Filter band	100–3000 Hz
Electrode montage	C_Z–A_1, C_Z–A_2
Number of channels	2
Number of sweeps	1500 or F_{SP}

RESULTS:

Presentation Rate:		7.7/second	27.7/second	57.7/second	77.7/second
Latency:	Wave I	_____	_____	_____	_____
	Wave III	_____	_____	_____	_____
	Wave V	_____	_____	_____	_____
	Waves I–III	_____	_____	_____	_____
	Waves III–V	_____	_____	_____	_____
	Waves I–V	_____	_____	_____	_____
Amplitude:	Wave I–I'	_____	_____	_____	_____
	Wave V–V'	_____	_____	_____	_____
	Wave V/I	_____	_____	_____	_____

NOTES: As rate is increased, the earlier components generally show an amplitude decrease. Absolute latencies increase more for the later components than the earlier components with increasing rate, resulting in an increase in the Waves I–V interwave interval. (See Figure 2–6.)

5. Comparison of Electrode Montages

In this exercise, two-channel ABRs will be recorded using click stimuli and three different electrode montages. Absolute latencies, interwave latencies, and amplitude will be determined.

Comparison of Electrode Montages

Parameter	Setup
Stimulus type	Click
Stimulus polarity	Condensation or rarefaction
Intensity	75 dB nHL
Presentation rate	27.7/second
Time base	12 ms
Filter band	100–3000 Hz
Electrode montage	C_z-A_1, C_z-A_2
	C_z-A_1, F_z-A_1
	C_z-A_1, C_z-C_7
Number of channels	2
Number of sweeps	1500 or F_{SP}

RESULTS:

Electrode Montage:		C_z-A_1, C_z-A_2	C_z-A_1, F_z-A_1	C_z-A_1, C_z-C_7
Latency:	Wave I	_____	_____	_____
	Wave III	_____	_____	_____
	Wave V	_____	_____	_____
	Waves I–III	_____	_____	_____
	Waves III–V	_____	_____	_____
	Waves I–V	_____	_____	_____
Amplitude:	Wave I–I'	_____	_____	_____
	Wave V–V'	_____	_____	_____
	Wave V/I	_____	_____	_____

NOTES: The electrode montages between the vertex or forehead and ears, used in the first and second recordings, will yield higher amplitude for the earlier components (e.g., Wave I). Changing the montage from C_z-A_1 to F_z-A_1, as in the second set of recordings, may result in a slight decrease in the amplitude of Wave V. In the third comparison, changing the montage from C_z-A_1 to C_z-C_7 should increase the amplitude of Wave V and may decrease the amplitude of Wave I.

6. Effects of Filter Settings

In this exercise, two-channel ABRs to clicks will be recorded using three different filter bands. Absolute latencies, interwave latencies, and amplitude will be determined.

Effects of Filter Settings

Parameter	Setup
Stimulus type	Click
Stimulus polarity	Condensation or rarefaction
Intensity	75 dB nHL
Presentation rate	27.7/second
Time base	12 ms
Filter band	*100–3000 Hz*
	30–3000 Hz
	30–1500 Hz
Electrode montage	$C_Z–A_1, C_Z–A_2$
Number of channels	2
Number of sweeps	1500 or F_{SP}

RESULTS:

Filter Setting:		100–3000 Hz	30–3000 Hz	30–1500 Hz
Latency:	Wave I	_____	_____	_____
	Wave III	_____	_____	_____
	Wave V	_____	_____	_____
	Waves I–III	_____	_____	_____
	Waves III–V	_____	_____	_____
	Waves I–V	_____	_____	_____
Amplitude:	Wave I–I'	_____	_____	_____
	Wave V–V'	_____	_____	_____
	Wave V/I	_____	_____	_____

NOTES: Changes in filter settings may affect the amplitude and latency of certain components of the ABR. Changing the low-frequency setting from 100 to 30 Hz increases the low-frequency energy in the response, which can be used in an attempt to accentuate the amplitude of Wave V. Narrowing the band pass of the filter can be used to reduce unrelated noise. Potential effects on amplitude and latency values should be kept in mind when comparing results to normative data. (See Figure 4–3.)

7. 500-Hz Toneburst ABR

In this exercise, a two-channel ABR will be recorded using 500-Hz tonebursts as the stimulus. Latencies of the primary peak will be determined as a function of stimulus intensity. These latencies can then be compared to normative data.

500-Hz Toneburst ABR

Parameter	Setup
Stimulus type	Toneburst
Stimulus frequency	500 Hz
Stimulus envelope	4 ms rise time
(2-0-2 cycles)	4 ms fall time
	0 ms plateau
Stimulus polarity	Condensation
Intensity	75, 55, 35 dB nHL
Presentation rate	39.1/second
Time base	20 ms
Filter band	30–1500 Hz
Electrode montage	C_Z–A_1, C_Z–A_2
Number of channels	2
Number of sweeps	1500

RESULTS:

		Left Ear	Right Ear
Latency:	___ dB nHL	_____	_____
	___ dB nHL	_____	_____
	___ dB nHL	_____	_____
	___ dB nHL	_____	_____
	___ dB nHL	_____	_____
	___ dB nHL	_____	_____

NOTES: ABRs to tonebursts at 500 Hz generally result in a single large peak. The primary purpose of testing is to determine the lowest level where a reliable response is obtained. The latency of the primary peak of the response can be determined and compared to normative data such as that published by Gorga et al. (1988). When the peak is rounded or contains several small "wavelets," the midpoint of the peak can be marked and compared to normative data. (See Figures 6–8 and 6–9.)

8. Bone-Conduction ABR

In this exercise, a two-channel ABR will be recorded using bone-conducted clicks at various intensities. Wave V latency and amplitude will be examined at each stimulus level in order to determine the threshold of the response.

Bone-Conduction ABR	
Parameter	**Setup**
Stimulus type	Click
Stimulus polarity	Alternating
Intensity	Near maximum, then decrease
Presentation rate	27.7/second
Time base	12 ms
Filter band	100–3000 Hz
Electrode montage	C_z–A_1, C_z–A_2
Number of channels	2
Number of sweeps	1500

RESULTS:

	Wave V Latency	V–V' Amplitude
___ dB nHL	_____	_____
___ dB nHL	_____	_____
___ dB nHL	_____	_____
___ dB nHL	_____	_____
___ dB nHL	_____	_____
___ dB nHL	_____	_____

NOTES: Bone-conducted ABRs generally do not show the clear five-wave complex observed when recording air-conducted ABRs at high intensities. This is due to the fact that the highest output from the bone-conduction oscillator is limited. Thus, bone-conduction ABRs will appear more like air-conduction ABRs obtained at lower intensities. The usual purpose of the bone-conduction ABR is to determine the lowest intensity where a reliable response can be recorded. Usually, only Wave V needs to be marked and compared to normative data. (See Figure 6–10.)

9. 40-Hz Response Using a 500-Hz Toneburst

In this exercise, a two-channel 40-Hz response will be recorded using a 500-Hz toneburst stimulus. Presence or absence of responses will be determined as a function of stimulus intensity and the threshold of the response identified.

40-Hz Response with 500-Hz Toneburst

Parameter	Setup
Stimulus type	Toneburst
Stimulus frequency	500 Hz
Stimulus envelope	4 ms rise time
(2-0-2 cycles)	4 ms fall time
	0 ms plateau
Stimulus polarity	Condensation
Intensity	75, 55, 35, 15 dB nHL
Presentation rate	39.1/second
Time base	100 ms
Filter band	5 (or 10)–100 Hz
Electrode montage	C_Z–A_1, C_Z–A_2
Number of channels	2
Number of sweeps	200
Number of runs	2 to 4

RESULTS:

Latency:		Peak 1	Peak 2	Peak 3	Peak 4
___ dB nHL		_____	_____	_____	_____
___ dB nHL		_____	_____	_____	_____
___ dB nHL		_____	_____	_____	_____
___ dB nHL		_____	_____	_____	_____
___ dB nHL		_____	_____	_____	_____

Amplitude:		Peak 1–1'	Peak 2–2'	Peak 3–3'	Peak 4–4'
___ dB nHL		_____	_____	_____	_____
___ dB nHL		_____	_____	_____	_____
___ dB nHL		_____	_____	_____	_____
___ dB nHL		_____	_____	_____	_____
___ dB nHL		_____	_____	_____	_____

NOTES: The 40-Hz response is characterized by a series of sinusoidal peaks that are approximately 25 ms apart. The latencies can be marked for each peak (either positive or negative) and then the interpeak differences calculated to determine if the peaks are separated by approximately 25 ms. The lowest intensity where a reliable 40-Hz response can be recorded denotes the threshold of the response. (See Figures 6–11 and 6–12.)

II. PROTOCOL PRACTICE

1. Neurological Application

SETUP:

1. Apply electrodes to C_Z, A_1, A_2, and ground.
2. Set up montages for a two-channel recording (C_Z–A_1, C_Z–A_2).

TEST:

1. Obtain ABRs for the right and left ears for 75 dB nHL (or appropriate intensity) at 7.7, 27.7, and 57.7 clicks per second.
2. Obtain two repetitions for each condition
3. At 7.7 per second, obtain at least one average using clicks of the opposite polarity.

INTERPRETATION:

1. Note the latencies for Waves I, III, and V.
2. Calculate the interwave latencies for Waves I–III, III–V, and I–V.
3. Compare responses to condensation and rarefaction clicks.
4. Compare Wave V latencies for each of the three stimulus rates.
5. Calculate Waves I–I' and V–V' amplitudes and determine the amplitude ratio.
6. Compare results to other audiological information.

2. Estimation of Hearing Sensitivity in Infants

SETUP:

1. Apply electrodes to F_Z, A_1 (or M_1), A_2 (or M_2), C_7, and ground.
2. Set up montages for a two-channel recording (F_Z–A_1 [or M_1] and F_Z–C_7 for left ear stimulation; F_Z–A_2 [or M_2] and F_Z–C_7 for right ear stimulation).
3. Use the contralateral ear electrode for ground (A_2 [or M_2] for left ear stimulation; A_1 [or M_1] for right ear stimulation).

TEST:

1. Obtain ABRs for air-conduction condensation clicks at 75, 55, 35, and 15 dB nHL for each ear at a presentation rate of 27.7 clicks per second. If no response is present when intensity is decreased, increase intensity by 10 dB. Obtain two repetitions at each intensity or use the F_{SP} estimation.
2. Obtain at least one average using rarefaction polarity clicks.

3. Obtain ABRs for air-conduction condensation 500-Hz tonebursts at 75, 55, and 35 dB nHL for each ear at a presentation rate of 27.7 clicks per second. If no response is present when intensity is decreased, increase intensity by 10 dB. Obtain two repetitions at each intensity.

4. Obtain ABRs for bone-conduction, alternating clicks at 45, 35, and 15 dB nHL for each ear at a presentation rate of 27.7 clicks per second. If no response is present when intensity is decreased, increase intensity by 10 dB. Obtain two repetitions at each intensity.

INTERPRETATION:

1. Note the latencies for Waves I, III, and V for clicks at 75 dB nHL (or another high intensity).
2. Calculate the interwave latencies for Waves I–III, III–V, and I–V at 75 dB nHL (or another high intensity).
3. Plot Wave V latency for each intensity on the infant latency-intensity function for air- and bone-conducted clicks. (See Figure 7–3.)
4. Compare responses to condensation and rarefaction clicks.
5. Compare toneburst latencies to a normative latency-intensity function for 500-Hz tonebursts.
6. Compare results to other audiological information.

3. Estimation of Hearing Sensitivity in Older Children or Adults

SETUP:

1. Apply electrodes to C_Z, A_1, A_2, and ground.
2. Set up montages for a two-channel recording (C_Z–A_1 and C_Z–A_2).

TEST:

1. Obtain ABRs for air-conduction condensation clicks at 75, 55, 35, and 15 dB nHL for each ear at a presentation rate of 27.7 clicks per second. If no response is present when intensity is decreased, increase intensity by 10 dB. Obtain two repetitions at each intensity or use F_{SP} estimation.
2. Obtain at least one average using rarefaction polarity clicks.
3. Obtain 40-Hz responses for 500-Hz tonebursts at 75, 55, 35, and 15 dB nHL for each ear at a presentation rate of 39.1 clicks per second. If no response is present when intensity is decreased, increase intensity by 10 dB. Obtain two repetitions at each intensity.
4. Obtain ABRs for bone-conduction alternating clicks at 45, 35, and 15 dB nHL for each ear at a presentation rate of 27.7 clicks per second. If no response is

present when intensity is decreased, increase intensity by 10 dB. Obtain two repetitions at each intensity.

INTERPRETATION:

1. Note the latencies for Waves I, III, and V for clicks at 75 dB nHL (or another high intensity).
2. Calculate the interwave latencies for Waves I–III, III–V, and I–V for 75-dB nHL clicks (or another high intensity).
3. Plot Wave V latency for each intensity on the adult latency-intensity function for air- and bone-conducted clicks. (See Figure A–1.)
4. Compare responses to condensation and rarefaction clicks.
5. Determine thresholds for the 40-Hz responses to 500-Hz tonebursts for each ear.
6. Compare results to other audiological information.

III. SKILL CHECKLIST

You should be able to:

_____ 1. Apply electrodes and check impedance.
_____ 2. Obtain an ABR for high-intensity condensation and rarefaction clicks.
_____ 3. Mark latencies for Waves I, III, and V and calculate interwave intervals.
_____ 4. Calculate Waves I–I' and V–V' amplitudes and determine the Waves V/I amplitude ratio.
_____ 5. Calculate changes in latency for Wave V with increases in stimulus rate.
_____ 6. Improve noisy responses.
_____ 7. Enhance Wave I amplitude.
_____ 8. Obtain an intensity series for air-conducted clicks and plot a Wave V latency-intensity function.
_____ 9. Obtain an intensity series for air-conducted 500-Hz tonebursts and plot a Wave V latency-intensity function.
_____ 10. Obtain an intensity series for bone-conducted clicks and plot a Wave V latency-intensity function.
_____ 11. Obtain an intensity series for the 40-Hz response using 500-Hz tonebursts.

Glossary

40-Hz response: An auditory evoked potential where the response waveform approximates the rate of stimulation.

Absolute latency: In auditory evoked potentials, the time in milliseconds from the occurrence of a stimulus to a peak in the waveform.

Action potential (AP): In auditory evoked potential measurements, the whole-nerve response of the eighth cranial nerve, which is a main component of the electrocochleogram and Wave I of the auditory brainstem response.

Air conduction: The transmission of sound, delivered via an earphone, through the outer and middle ear to the cochlea.

Amplitude: In auditory evoked potential measurements, the magnitude of the response. The scale used in the auditory brainstem response is microvolts.

Artifact: Any unwanted signal included in a response that is not related to the desired neural response.

Auditory brainstem response (ABR): An auditory evoked potential that represents neural activity from the eighth cranial nerve and auditory pathways of the brainstem. Other terms used include brainstem auditory evoked potential (BAEP) and brainstem auditory evoked response (BAER).

Auditory evoked potential (AEP): Electrophysiological responses representing neural responses of auditory pathways from the eighth cranial nerve to the cortex.

Bone conduction: Transmission of sound to the cochlea via vibration of the skull.

Bone-conducted click: A short-duration pulse delivered via a bone-conduction oscillator.

Brainstem: Portion of the brain made up of the medulla, pons, and midbrain, located between the spinal cord and the diencephalon (which lies between the brainstem and the cerebral hemispheres).

CAPD: Central auditory processing disorder. An impairment in the ability of the central auditory system to process and utilize auditory signals.

Central auditory nervous system (CANS): Portion of the nervous system composed of auditory pathways from the eighth cranial nerve through the cerebral hemispheres.

Click: A rapid onset, short duration, broad-band sound produced by delivering an electrical pulse to a transducer.

CNS: Central nervous system. That portion of the nervous system to which sensory impulses and from which motor impulses are transmitted.

Cochlear microphonic (CM): Alternating-current electrical potentials from the hair cells of the cochlea that resemble the input signal.

Cochlear potentials (CPs): Bioelectric potentials generated in the cochlea.

Common mode rejection (CMR): A noise rejection strategy used in recording evoked potentials where noise that is identical, or common, at two electrodes is subtracted by a differential amplifier.

Computer averaging: Signal averaging with a computer.

Computed tomography (CT): Also referred to as computerized axial tomography (CAT). A radiological procedure that produces images of the anatomy by acquiring sectional radiographs of specified areas presented as a computer image.

Coronal plane: A midline division of body that divides the front from the back.

Cortex: Sheets of gray matter covering the cerebral hemispheres.

Cortical potential or response: Long-latency evoked potentials generated from neural sources in the cerebrum.

Cross-check principle: A principle in audiometry that states that the results of any single audiometric test cannot be considered valid without independent verification from another test.

Decibel (dB): Unit of sound intensity, based on the ratio of one intensity to a reference intensity, derived from the formula: $10 \log_{10} (I_O/I_{REF})$.

Demyelinating disease: Disease process that causes scattered patches of demyelination of white matter throughout the central nervous system.

Differential amplifier: An amplifier used in evoked potential measurement to reduce unwanted noise. The voltage from one electrode is inverted and then added to the voltage of another electrode.

Diffuse lesions: Lesions that are not localized or do not have defined limitation.

Distortion product otoacoustic emissions (DPOAEs): Used clinically, otoacoustic emissions that represent the cubic distortion product (2f1–f2) occurring from simultaneous presentation of combinations of two pure tones (f1 and f2).

Electrical field: An area surrounding a generator from which the spread of electrical activity occurs.

Electrocochleography (ECochG): A method of recording transient auditory evoked potentials, including the cochlear microphonic, summating potential, and eighth nerve action potential, from the cochlea and eighth nerve using an electrode at the promontory or in the ear canal.

Electrode: A specialized metal plate through which electrical stimuli are measured from or applied to the body.

Electroencephalography (EEG): A method of recording electrical potentials from scalp electrodes.

Endogenous response: In evoked potentials, a response that changes more according to internal factors, such as perception of the event, than to external factors.

Envelope: In acoustics, the representation of the onset, plateau, and offset times of a waveform. Onset and offset characteristics may be defined by various mathematical functions, such as cosine-square, Hamming, and Blackmann.

Evoked otoacoustic emissions (EOAEs): Otoacoustic emissions that occur in response to acoustic stimulation.

Evoked potential (EP): Electrical activity occurring in the peripheral and central nervous system in response to stimulation.

Exogenous response: In evoked potentials, a response that changes according to the dimensions of an external event.

Fall time: The time required for a gated signal to decrease from its maximum intensity to a specified percentage of its maximum amplitude. Also referred to as decay time.

Far-field: A *far-field* recording occurs when recording electrodes are at a distance from the source of the electrical potential. An example is the auditory brainstem response.

Frequency following response (FFR): A short-latency auditory evoked potential of the same frequency as the response-eliciting stimulus.

Frequency selectivity: The ability to discriminate among sounds of different frequencies.

F_{SP}: An algorithm used to estimate the statistical likelihood of the presence of a response, based on the F distribution of the variance of the response divided by the variance of a single point (SP) in time across successive samples.

Functional disorder: Dysfunction in the absence of any known organic cause.

Glioma: A tumor composed of neuroglia, the supporting structure of nervous tissue.

Glycerin test: A diagnostic test used for Ménière's disease in which auditory function is assessed before and after ingestion of glycerin.

Ground electrode: An electrode that is placed on the patient, frequently at F_{PZ}, that attaches the patient to ground. Also referred to as a common electrode.

Hearing level (HL): The decibel threshold of an individual relative to the average threshold of normal young adults. Used interchangeably with *hearing threshold level* (HTL).

Hearing screening: A method of separating individuals with normal hearing from individuals with abnormal hearing.

Hearing sensitivity: Capacity of the auditory system to detect a stimulus, generally determined by measuring responses to stimuli presented at progressively lower intensities.

Hearing threshold level (HTL): The threshold of an individual relative to the average threshold of normal young adults. Used interchangeably with *hearing level* (HL).

Immittance: A term representing energy flow through the middle ear, including admittance, compliance, conductance, impedance, reactance, resistance, and susceptance.

Inion: The most prominent point of the external occipital protuburance, located at the back of the head.

Interwave latency: The difference, in milliseconds, between two peaks of an auditory evoked potential.

Intraoperative monitoring: Continuous assessment of neural integrity during surgical procedures.

Late cortical responses: Long-latency auditory evoked potentials that may include the vertex response (N1–P2), P300, mismatch negativity (MMN), and other responses from the auditory pathways of the cerebrum.

Latency: The time interval between two events, such as a stimulus and a response.

Magnetic resonance imaging (MRI): A diagnostic radiological procedure used to image anatomy by placing the body in a magnetic field and presenting radiofrequency pulses.

Masking level difference (MLD): Improvement in binaural masked thresholds when the noise phase relationship is altered as compared to stimuli that are identical in both ears.

Maximum length sequence (MLS): A signal-processing technique that permits presentation of stimuli at rapid rates and subsequent deconvolution of interleaved patterns into their component responses.

Meningioma: A slow-growing, usually vascular tumor that occurs mainly along the meningeal vessels and superior longitudinal sinus.

Microvolt (μV): 10^{-6} volts, or one millionth of a volt.

Middle ear muscle reflexes (MEMRs): Reflexive contraction of the stapedius and tensor tympani muscles of the middle ear in response to loud sound.

Middle latency response (MLR): An auditory evoked potential representing neural activity from, at least in part, auditory radiations from the thalamus to the cortex and the primary auditory cortex.

Millivolt (mV): 10^{-3} volts, or one thousandth of a volt.

Mismatch negativity (MMN): A late auditory evoked potential occurring in the 100- to 200-ms latency range that represents neural activity obtained by utilizing combinations of auditory stimuli presented in an oddball paradigm.

Montage: The electrode positions on the scalp used to record electrical responses. Usually referred to the 10-20 International Standard (Jasper, 1958).

Morphology: The *qualitative* features of an evoked potential. It considers the "noisiness" of the recording, the "smoothness" of the recording, the replicability of the recording, and how the recording compares to an ideal recording.

Multiple sclerosis: Demyelinating disease in which plaques form throughout the white matter, resulting in diffuse neurological symptoms.

Muscle artifact: Muscle potentials that occur to random muscle activity or sensory stimulation in the same time frame as the desired response.

Nasion: Depression at the root of the nose that indicates the position of the frontonasal suture.

Near-field: A *near-field* recording is situated close to the source of an electrical potential. An example is direct eighth nerve recording.

Neural synchrony: The ability of a group of neurons to activate simultaneously.

Neurilemmoma: A benign tumor of a peripheral nerve sheath. Also referred to as a neurinoma, neuroma, or Schwannoma.

Neuron: The basic unit of the nervous system, consisting of an axon, cell body, and dendrites, which transmit information, usually in the form of nerve impulses.

Neuropathy: A disorder of the nervous system.

nHL: The hearing level for a click relative to the average threshold of a group of normal-hearing young adults.

Nyquist frequency: The frequency equal to one half of the analog-to-digital sampling rate. This is the highest frequency that can be sampled without aliasing.

Ohms (Ω): Units of resistance of a conductor to electrical or other forms of energy.

Otoacoustic emissions (OAEs): Low-level sounds emitted by the normal cochlea.

P300 response: A late auditory evoked potential occurring in the 300-ms latency range that represents neural activity obtained by utilizing combinations of auditory stimuli presented in an oddball paradigm.

Peak: An amplitude measurement made from an average baseline to a positive peak or negative peak (i.e., trough).

Peak-to-peak amplitude: An amplitude measurement made from a positive peak to a negative peak representing the two extremes of the waveform.

Peak sound pressure (peak SP or pSP): The maximum physical intensity of a short-duration stimulus.

PIPB function: Performance-intensity (PI) function for phonetically balanced (PB) word lists.

PIPB rollover: Decrease in speech recognition at high intensity levels, consistent with a retrocochlear lesion.

Plateau: The time that a signal is at its maximum intensity.

Pulse: A brief electrical signal, usually a square wave.

Rise time: The time required for a gated signal to proceed from baseline to a specified percentage of its maximum amplitude.

Sagittal plane: A midline division of the body that divides the left and right sides of the body.

Sensation level (SL): The intensity of a sound above an individual's threshold for that sound.

Signal averaging: A technique of averaging of successive samples of electro-encephalographic activity time-locked to a stimulus in order to reduce unrelated signals and thus improve the signal-to-noise ratio.

SN_{10} response: Slow negative auditory evoked response occurring at approximately 10 ms after signal onset, usually acquired using low-frequency tone-burst stimuli.

Space-occupying lesion: A neoplasm that exerts its influence by impinging on neural tissues.

Steady state evoked potential (SSEP): An auditory evoked potential where the response waveform approximates the rate of stimulation. Also referred to as SSR.

Steady state response (SSR): An auditory evoked potential where the response waveform approximates the rate of stimulation. Also referred to as SSEP.

Summating potential (SP): A direct-current electrical potential of cochlear origin that can be measured using electrocochleography.

Toneburst: Signals having a rise time, plateau time, and fall or decay time of sufficient duration to be perceived as having tonal quality.

Transducer: A device that converts one form of energy to another, such as an earphone that converts electrical to acoustic energy.

Tumor: An abnormal growth of tissue resulting from an excessively rapid proliferation of cells.

Tympanogram: A graph of middle ear immittance as a function of the amount of air pressure delivered to the ear canal.

Vertex: The summit or top of the head.

VIIIth nerve: The eighth cranial nerve, known as the vestibulocochlear nerve, consisting of vestibular and cochlear branches.

References

Allison, T., Wood, C. C., & Goff, W. R. (1983). Brain stem auditory, pattern-reversal visual, and short-latency somatosensory evoked potentials: Latencies in relation to age, sex, and brain and body size. *Electroencephalography and Clinical Neurophysiology, 55,* 619–636.

Aoyagi, M., Yokota, M., Nakamura, T., Tojima, H., Kim, Y., Suzuki, Y., Koike, Y., & Nakai, O. (1994). Hearing preservation and improvement of auditory brainstem response findings after acoustic neuroma surgery. *Acta Oto-Laryngologica, Suppl. 511,* 40–46.

Arezzo, J., Legatt, A. D., & Vaughan, H. G., Jr. (1979). Topography and intracranial sources of somatosensory evoked potentials in the monkey: I. Early components. *Electroencephalography and Clinical Neurophysiology, 46,* 155–172.

Arnold, J. E., & Bender, D. R. (1983). BSER abnormalities in a multiple sclerosis patient with normal peripheral hearing acuity. *American Journal of Otology, 4,* 235–237.

Barrs, D. M., Brackmann, D. E., Olson, J. E., & House, W. F. (1985). Changing concepts of acoustic tumor diagnosis. *Archives of Otolaryngology, 111,* 17–21.

Bauch, C. D., & Olsen, W. (1986). The effect of 2000–4000 Hz hearing sensitivity on ABR results. *Ear and Hearing, 7,* 314–317.

Bauch, C. D., & Olsen, W. (1987). Average 2000 to 4000 Hz hearing sensitivity and ABR results. *Ear and Hearing, 8,* 184.

Bauch, C. D., Olsen, W., & Pool, A. F. (1996). ABR indices: Sensitivity, specificity, and tumor size. *American Journal of Audiology, 5,* 97–104.

Bauch, C. D., Rose, D. E., & Harner, S. G. (1980). Brainstem responses to tone pip and click stimuli. *Ear and Hearing, 1,* 181–184.

Bauch, C. D., Rose, D. E., & Harner, S. G. (1982). Auditory brain stem response results from 255 patients with suspected retrocochlear involvement. *Ear and Hearing, 3,* 83–86.

Beagley, H., & Sheldrake, J. (1978). Differences in brainstem response latency with age and sex. *British Journal of Audiology, 12,* 69–77.

Beattie, R. C., Garcia, E., & Johnson, A. (1996). Frequency-specific auditory brainstem responses in adults with sensorineural hearing loss. *Audiology, 35,* 194–203.

Beattie, R. C., & Kennedy, K. M. (1992). Auditory brainstem response to tone bursts in quiet, notch noise, highpass noise, and broadband noise. *Journal of the American Academy of Audiology, 3,* 349–360.

Beattie, R. C., Moretti, M., & Warren, V. (1984). Effects of rise-fall time, frequency, and intensity on the early/middle evoked response. *Journal of Speech and Hearing Disorders, 49,* 114–127.

Beattie, R. C., Thielen, K. M., & Franzone, D. L. (1994). Effects of signal-to-noise ratio on the auditory brainstem response to tone bursts in notch noise and broadband noise. *Scandinavian Audiology, 23,* 47–56.

Berlin, C. I. (1996). The role of infant hearing screening in health care. *Seminars in Hearing, 17,* 115–124.

Berlin, C. I., Bordelon, J., St. John, P., Wilensky, D., Hurley, A., Kluka, E., & Hood, L. J. (1998). Reversing click polarity may uncover auditory neuropathy in infants. *Ear and Hearing, 19,* 37–47.

Berlin, C. I., Hood, L. J., Cecola, R. P., Jackson, D. F., & Szabo, P. (1993). Does Type I afferent neuron dysfunction reveal itself through lack of efferent suppression? *Hearing Research, 65,* 40–50.

Berlin, C. I., Hood, L. J., Hurley, A., & Wen, H. (1994). Contralateral suppression of otoacoustic emissions: An index of the function of the medial olivocochlear system. *Otolaryngology—Head and Neck Surgery, 100,* 3–21.

Berlin, C. I., & Shearer, P. S. (1984). *Long-term follow-up of brainstem evoked response and electrocochleography.* Paper presented at Society for Ear, Nose and Throat Advances in Children, New Orleans, LA.

Berlin, C. I., Wexler, K. F., Jerger, J. F., Halperin, H. R., & Smith, S. (1978). Superior ultra-audiometric hearing: A new type of hearing loss which correlates highly with unusually good speech in the "profoundly deaf." *Otolaryngology, 86,* 111–116.

Blegvad, B. (1975). Binaural summation of surface recorded electrocochleographic responses in normal hearing subjects. *Scandinavian Audiology, 4,* 233–238.

Borg, E., & Lofqvist, L. (1982). Auditory brainstem response (ABR) to rarefaction and condensation clicks in normal and abnormal ears. *Scandinavian Audiology, 11,* 227–235.

Brantberg, K. (1996). Easily applied ear canal electrodes improve the diagnostic potential of auditory brainstem response. *Scandinavian Audiology, 25,* 147–152.

Campbell, K. C. M., & Brady, B. A. (1995). Comparison of 1000-Hz toneburst and click stimuli in otoneurologic ABR. *American Journal of Audiology, 4,* 55–60.

Cashman, M. Z., Stanton, S. G., Sagle, C., & Barber, H. O. (1993). The effect of hearing loss on ABR interpretation: Use of a correction factor. *Scandinavian Audiology, 22,* 153–158.

Chandrasekhar, S. S., Brackmann, D. E., & Devgan, K. K. (1996). Utility of auditory brainstem response audiometry in diagnosis of acoustic neuromas. *American Journal of Otology, 16,* 63–67.

Chiappa, K. H., Gladstone, K. J., & Young, R. R. (1979). Brainstem auditory evoked responses. *Archives of Neurology, 36,* 81–87.

Chiappa, K. H., Harrison, J. L., Brooks, E. B., & Young, R. (1980). Brainstem auditory evoked responses in 200 patients with multiple sclerosis. *Annals of Neurology, 7,* 135–143.

Chu, N., Squires, K., & Starr, A. (1978). Auditory brainstem potentials in chronic ethanol intoxication and alcohol withdrawal. *Archives of Neurology, 35,* 596–602.

Clemis, J. D., & McGee, T. (1979). Brain stem electric response audiometry in the differential diagnosis of acoustic tumors. *Laryngoscope, 89,* 31–42.

Clemis, J. D., & Mitchell, C. (1977). Electrocochleography and brain stem responses used in the diagnosis of tumors. *Journal of Otolaryngology, 6,* 447–459.

Coats, A. C. (1978). Human auditory nerve action potentials and brain stem evoked responses. *Archives of Otolaryngology, 104,* 709–717.

Coats, A. C. (1981). The summating potential and Ménière's disease: I. Summating potential amplitude in Ménière and non-Ménière ears. *Archives of Otolaryngology, 103,* 199–208.

Coats, A. C., & Martin, J. L. (1977). Human auditory nerve action potentials and brain stem evoked responses: Effects of audiogram shape and lesion location. *Archives of Otolaryngology, 103,* 605–622.

Cohen, N. L., Lewis, W. S., & Ransohoff, J. (1993). Hearing preservation in cerebellopontine angle tumor surgery: The NYU experience 1974–1991. *American Journal of Otology, 14,* 423–433.

Cohen, L. T., Rickards, F. W., & Clark, G. M. (1991). A comparison of steady-state evoked potentials to modulated tones in awake and sleeping humans. *Journal of the Acoustical Society of America, 90,* 2467–2479.

Cone-Wesson, B., & Ramirez, G. M. (1997). Hearing sensitivity in newborns estimated from ABRs to bone-conducted sounds. *Journal of the American Academy of Audiology, 8,* 299–307.

Cox, C., Hack, M., & Metz, D. (1981). Brainstem-evoked response audiometry: Normative data from the preterm infant. *Audiology, 20,* 53–64.

Creel, D., Boxer, L. A., & Fauci, A. S. (1983). Visual and auditory anomalies in Chediak-Higashi syndrome. *Electroencephalography and Clinical Neurophysiology, 55,* 252–257.

Davis, H. (1976). Principles of electric response audiometry. *Annals of Otology, Rhinology and Laryngology, Suppl. 28,* 4–96.

Davis, H., & Hirsh, S. K. (1979). A slow brain stem response for low-frequency audiometry. *Audiology, 18,* 445–461.

Davis, H., Hirsh, S. K., & Turpin, L. L. (1983). Possible utility of middle latency responses in electric response audiometry. *Advances in Otology, Rhinology and Laryngology, 31,* 208–216.

Davis, H., Hirsh, S. K., Turpin, L. L., & Peacock, M. E. (1985). Threshold sensitivity and frequency specificity in ABR audiometry. *Audiology, 24,* 54–70.

Davis, P. A. (1939). Effects of acoustic stimuli on the waking human brain. *Journal of Neurophysiology, 2,* 494–499.

De Donato, G., Russo, A., Taibah, A., Saleh, E., & Sanna, M. (1995). Incidence of normal hearing in acoustic neuroma. *Acta Otorhinolaryngologica Italica, 15,* 73–79.

Deltenre, P., Mansbach, A., Bozet, C., Clercx, A., & Hecox, K. (1997). Auditory neuropathy: A report on three cases with early onsets and major neonatal illnesses. *Electroencephalography and Clinical Neurophysiology, 104,* 17–22.

Djupesland, G., Flottorp, G., Modalsli, B., Tvete, O., & Sortland, O. (1981). Acoustic brain stem response in diagnosis of acoustic neuroma. *Scandinavian Audiology, 10* (Suppl. 13), 109–112.

Dobie, R. A., & Berlin, C. I. (1979). Binaural interaction in brainstem-evoked responses. *Archives of Otolaryngology, 105,* 391–398.

Dobie, R. A., & Norton, S. J. (1980). Binaural interaction in human auditory evoked potentials. *Electroencephalography and Clinical Neurophysiology, 49,* 303–313.

Don, M., Allen, A. R., & Starr, A. (1977). Effect of click rate on the latency of auditory brain stem responses in humans. *Annals of Otolaryngology, 86,* 186–195.

Don, M., & Eggermont, J. J. (1978). Analysis of the click-evoked brainstem potentials in man using high-pass noise masking. *Journal of the Acoustical Society of America, 63,* 1084–1092.

Don, M., Eggermont, J. J., & Brackmann, D. E. (1979). Reconstruction of the audiogram using brain stem responses and high-pass masking noise. *Annals of Otology, Rhinology and Laryngology, 88* (Suppl. 57), 1–20.

Don, M., & Elberling, C. (1996). Use of quantitative measures of auditory brain-stem response peak amplitude and residual background noise in the decision to stop averaging. *Journal of the Acoustical Society of America, 99,* 491–499.

Don, M., Elberling, C., & Waring, M. (1984). Objective detection of averaged auditory brainstem responses. *Scandinavian Audiology, 13,* 219–228.

Don, M., Ponton, C. W., Eggermont, J. J., & Masuda, A. (1994). Auditory brainstem response (ABR) peak amplitude variability reflects individual differences in cochlear response times. *Journal of the Acoustical Society of America, 96,* 3476–3491.

Dornhoffer, J. L., Helms, J., & Hoehmann, D. H. (1995). Hearing preservation in acoustic tumor surgery: Results and prognostic factors. *Laryngoscope, 105,* 184–187.

Durrant, J. D., & Fowler, C. G. (1996). ABR protocols for dealing with asymmetric hearing loss. *American Journal of Audiology, 5,* 5–6.

Eggermont, J., Don, M., & Brackmann, D. (1980). Electrocochleography and brainstem electric responses in patients with pontine angle tumors. *Annals of Otology, Rhinology and Laryngology, Suppl. 89,* 1–19.

Elberling, C., & Don, M. (1984). Quality estimation of averaged auditory brainstem responses. *Scandinavian Audiology, 13,* 187–197.

Elberling, C., & Don, M. (1987). Threshold characteristics of the human auditory brain stem response. *Journal of the Acoustical Society of America, 81,* 115–121.

Elberling, C., & Parbo, J. (1987). Reference data for ABRs in retrocochlear disease. *Scandinavian Audiology, 16,* 49–55.

Eldredge, L., & Salamy, A. (1996). Functional auditory development in preterm and full term infants. *Early Human Development, 45,* 215–228.

Evans, J., Webster, D., & Cullen, J. K., Jr. (1983). Auditory brainstem responses in neonatally sound-deprived CBA/J mice. *Hearing Research, 10,* 269–277.

Eysholdt, U., & Schreiner, C. (1982). Maximum length sequences—a fast method for measuring brainstem evoked responses. *Audiology, 21,* 242–250.

Fausti, S. A., Frey, R. H., Henry, J. A., Olson, D. J., & Schaffer, H. I. (1993). High-frequency techniques and instrumentation for early detection of ototoxicity. *Journal of Rehabilitation Research and Development, 30,* 333–341.

Fausti, S. A., Mitchell, C. R., Frey, R. H., Henry, J. A., & O'Connor, J. L. (1994). Multiple-stimulus method for rapid collection of auditory brainstem responses using high-frequency (> or = 8 kHz) tone bursts. *Journal of the American Academy of Audiology, 5,* 119–126.

Fausti, S. A., Olsen, D. J., Frey, R. H., Henry, J. A., & Schaffer, H. I. (1993). High-frequency tone burst ABR latency-intensity functions. *Scandinavian Audiology, 22,* 25–33.

Fausti, S. A., Olson, D. J., Frey, R. H., Henry, J. A., Schaffer, H. I., & Phillips, D. S. (1995). High-frequency toneburst-evoked ABR latency-intensity functions in sensorineural hearing-impaired humans. *Scandinavian Audiology, 24,* 19–25.

Ferguson, M. A., Smith, P. A., Lutman, M. E., Mason, S. M., Coles, R. R., & Gibbon, K. P. (1996). Efficiency of tests used to screen for cerebello-pontine angle tumours: A prospective study. *British Journal of Audiology, 30,* 159–176.

Ferraro, J., & Ferguson, R. (1989). Tympanic ECochG and conventional ABR: A combined approach for the identification of wave I and the I–V interwave interval. *Ear and Hearing, 10,* 161–166.

Finitzo-Hieber, T., Hecox, K., & Cone, B. (1979). Brain stem auditory evoked potentials in patients with congenital atresia. *Laryngoscope, 89,* 1151–1158.

Fowler, C. G., & Noffsinger, D. (1983). Effects of stimulus repetition rate and frequency on the auditory brainstem response in normal, cochlear-impaired, and VIII nerve/brainstem-impaired subjects. *Journal of Speech and Hearing Research, 26,* 560–567.

Foxe, J. J., & Stapells, D. R. (1993). Normal infant and adult auditory brainstem responses to bone-conducted tones. *Audiology, 32,* 95–109.

Fria, T., & Sabo, D. (1980). Auditory brainstem responses in children with otitis media with effusion. *Annals of Otology, Rhinology and Laryngology, Suppl. 68,* 200–206.

Fujikawa, S., & Weber, B. (1977). Effect of increased stimulus rate on brain stem electric response audiometry as a function of age. *Journal of the American Audiology Society, 3,* 147–150.

Galambos, R., & Hecox, K. E. (1978). Clinical applications of the auditory brain stem response. *Otolaryngologic Clinics of North America, 11,* 709–722.

Galambos, R., Hicks, G. E., & Wilson, M. J. (1982). Hearing loss in graduates of a tertiary intensive care nursery. *Ear and Hearing, 3,* 87–90.

Galambos, R., Hicks, G. E., & Wilson, M. J. (1984). The auditory brain stem response reliably predicts hearing loss in graduates of a tertiary intensive care nursery. *Ear and Hearing, 5,* 254–260.

Galambos, R., Makeig, S., & Talmachoff, P. J. (1981). A 40-Hz auditory potential recorded from the human scalp. *Proceedings of the National Academy of Sciences, 78,* 2643–2647.

Galambos, R., Wilson, M. J., & Silva, P. D. (1994). Identifying hearing loss in the intensive care nursery: A 20-year summary. *Journal of the American Academy of Audiology, 5,* 151–162.

Gardi, J. N., & Berlin, C. I. (1981). Binaural interaction components. *Archives of Otolaryngology, 107,* 164–168.

Gawal, M., Das, P., Vincent, S., & Rose, F. (1981). Visual and auditory evoked responses in patients with Parkinson's disease. *Journal of Neurology, Neurosurgery, and Psychiatry, 44,* 227–232.

Geisler, C. D., Frishkopf, L. S., & Rosenblith, W. A. (1958). Extracranial responses to acoustic clicks in man. *Science, 128,* 1210–1211.

Glasscock, M. E., Jackson, C. G., Josey, A. F., Dickins, R. E., & Wiet, R. J. (1979). Brain stem evoked response audiometry in a clinical practice. *Laryngoscope, 89,* 1021–1035.

Gordon, M. L., & Cohen, N. L. (1995). Efficacy of auditory brainstem response as a screening test for small acoustic neuromas. *American Journal of Otology, 16,* 136–139.

Gorga, M. P., Kaminski, J. R., & Beauchaine, K. A. (1991). Effects of stimulus phase on the latency of the auditory brainstem response. *Journal of the American Academy of Audiology, 2,* 1–6.

Gorga, M. P., Kaminski, J. R., Beauchaine, K. L., & Bergman, B. M. (1993). A comparison of auditory brain stem response thresholds and latencies elicited by air- and bone-conducted stimuli. *Ear and Hearing, 14,* 85–94.

Gorga, M. P., Kaminski, J. R., Beauchaine, K. A., & Jesteadt, W. (1988). Auditory brainstem responses to tone bursts in normally hearing subjects. *Journal of Speech and Hearing Research, 31,* 87–97.

Gorga, M. P., Kaminski, J. R., Beauchaine, K. A., & Schulte, L. (1992). Auditory brainstem responses elicited by 1000-Hz tone bursts in patients with sensorineural hearing loss. *Journal of the American Academy of Audiology, 3,* 159–165.

Gorga, M. P., Reiland, J. K., Beauchaine, K. A., Worthington, D. W., & Jesteadt, W. (1987). Auditory brainstem responses from graduates of an intensive care nursery: Normal patterns of response. *Journal of Speech and Hearing Research, 30,* 311–318.

Gorga, M. P., Stelmachowicz, P. G., Barlow, S. M., & Brookhouser, P. E. (1995). Case of recurrent, reversible, sudden sensorineural hearing loss in a child. *Journal of the American Academy of Audiology, 6,* 163–172.

Guerit, J. M., Mahieu, P., Houben-Giurgea, S., & Herbay, S. (1981). The influence of ototoxic drugs on brainstem auditory evoked potentials in man. *Archives of Oto-Rhino-Laryngology (Berlin), 233,* 189–199.

Hall, J. W., III. (1992). *Handbook of auditory evoked responses.* Boston: Allyn & Bacon.

Hall, J. W., & Grose, J. H. (1993). The effect of otitis media with effusion on the masking-level difference and the auditory brainstem response. *Journal of Speech and Hearing Research, 36,* 210–217.

Hall, J. W., III, & Mackey-Hargadine, J. (1984). Auditory evoked responses in severe head injury. *Seminars in Hearing, 5,* 313–336.

Hannley, M., Jerger, J., & Rivera, V. (1983). Relationships among auditory brainstem responses, masking level differences and the acoustic reflex in multiple sclerosis. *Audiology, 22,* 20–33.

Harker, L. A., Hosick, E., Voots, R. J., & Mendel, M. I. (1977). Influence of succinylcholine on middle-component auditory evoked potentials. *Archives of Otolaryngology, 103,* 133–137.

Harner, S. G., Harper, C. M., Beatty, C. W., Litchy, W. J., & Ebersold, M. J. (1996). Far-field auditory brainstem response in neurotologic surgery. *American Journal of Otology, 17,* 150–153.

Hawes, M. D., & Greenberg, H. J. (1981). Slow brain stem responses (SN_{10}) to tone pips in normally hearing newborns and adults. *Audiology, 20,* 113–122.

Hayes, D., & Jerger, J. (1981). Patterns of acoustic reflex and auditory brainstem response abnormality. *Acta Otolaryngologica, 92,* 199–209.

Hecox, K. E., & Cone, B. (1981). Prognostic importance of brainstem auditory evoked responses after asphyxia. *Neurology, 31,* 1429–1434.

Hecox, K. E., Cone, B., & Blaw, M. E. (1981). Brainstem auditory evoked response in the diagnosis of pediatric neurological diseases. *Neurology, 31,* 832–839.

Hecox, K. E., & Galambos, R. (1974). Brain stem auditory evoked responses in human infants and adults. *Archives of Otolaryngology, 99,* 30–33.

Hecox, K. E., Squires, N., & Galambos, R. (1976). Brainstem auditory evoked responses in man: I. Effect of stimulus rise-fall time and duration. *Journal of the Acoustical Society of America, 60,* 1187–1192.

Hood, L. J., & Berlin, C. I. (1986). *Auditory evoked potentials.* Austin, TX: Pro-Ed Publishers.

Hood, L. J., Berlin, C. I., & Allen, P. (1994). Cortical deafness: A longitudinal study. *Journal of the American Academy of Audiology, 5,* 330–342.

Hood, L. J., & Morehouse, C. R. (1985). Clinical application of insert earphones in auditory brainstem response testing. *Asha, 27,* 74.

Hooks, R. G., & Weber, B. A. (1984). Auditory brain stem responses of premature infants to bone-conducted stimuli: A feasibility study. *Ear and Hearing, 5,* 42–46.

Hosford-Dunn, H., Runge, C. A., Hillel, A., & Johnson, S. J. (1983). Auditory brain stem response testing in infants with collapsed ear canals. *Ear and Hearing, 4,* 258–260.

House, J. W., & Brackmann, D. E. (1979). Brainstem audiometry in neurotologic diagnosis. *Archives of Otolaryngology, 105,* 305–309.

Humes, L. E., & Ochs, M. G. (1982). Use of contralateral masking in the measurement of the auditory brainstem response. *Journal of Speech and Hearing Research, 25,* 528–535.

Hyde, M. L., Matsumoto, N., & Alberti, P. W. (1987). The normative basis for click and frequency-specific BERA in high-risk infants. *Acta Otolaryngologica (Stockholm), 103,* 602–611.

Hyde, M. L., Stephens, S. D. G., & Thornton, A. R. D. (1976). Stimulus repetition rate and the early brainstem responses. *British Journal of Audiology, 10,* 41–50.

Jacobson, G. P., Newman, C. W., Monsell, E., & Wharton, J. A. (1993). False negative auditory brainstem response findings in vestibular schwannoma: Case reports. *Journal of the American Academy of Audiology, 4,* 355–359.

Jacobson, J. T. (Ed.). (1994). *Principles and applications in auditory evoked potentials.* Boston: Allyn & Bacon.

Jacobson, J. T., & Hecox, K. E. (1982). Auditory brainstem response audiometry: Application and limitations to pediatric assessment. *Asha, 24,* 712.

Jacobson, J. T., Jacobson, C. A., & Spahr, R. C. (1990). Automated and conventional ABR screening techniques in high-risk infants. *Journal of the American Academy of Audiology, 1,* 187–195.

Jacobson, J. T., & Morehouse, C. R. (1984). A comparison of auditory brain stem response and behavioral screening in risk and normal newborn infants. *Ear and Hearing, 5,* 247–253.

Jacobson, J. T., Morehouse, C. R., & Johnson, M. J. (1982). Strategies for infant auditory brain stem response assessment. *Ear and Hearing, 3,* 263–270.

Japaridze, G., Kvernadze, D., Geladze, T., & Kevanishvili, Z. (1993). Effects of carbamazepine on auditory brainstem response, middle-latency response, and slow cortical potential in epileptic patients. *Epilepsia, 34,* 1105–1109.

Jasper, H. H. (1958). The ten-twenty electrode system of the International Federation. *Electroencephalography and Clinical Neurophysiology, 10,* 371–375.

Jerger, J., & Hall, J. (1980). Effects of age and sex on auditory brainstem response. *Archives of Otolaryngology, 106,* 387–391.

Jerger, J., Hayes, D., & Jordan, C. (1980). Clinical experience with auditory brainstem response audiometry in pediatric assessment. *Ear and Hearing, 1,* 19–25.

Jerger, J., & Johnson, K. (1988). Interactions of age, gender, and sensorineural hearing loss on ABR latency. *Ear and Hearing, 9,* 168–176.

Jerger, J., & Mauldin, L. (1978). Prediction of sensori-neural hearing level from the brain stem evoked response. *Archives of Otolaryngology, 104,* 454–461.

Jerger, J., Mauldin, L., & Anthony, L. (1978). Brain-stem evoked response audiometry in neuro-otologic evaluation. *Audiology and Hearing Education, 4,* 17–18, 20, 24.

Jerger, J., Neely, J. G., & Jerger, S. (1980). Speech, impedance, and auditory brainstem response audiometry in brainstem tumors. *Archives of Otolaryngology, 106,* 218–223.

Jerger, J., Oliver, T. A., Chmiel, R. A., & Rivera, V. M. (1986). Patterns of auditory abnormality in multiple sclerosis. *Audiology, 25,* 193–209.

Jerger, J., Oliver, T., & Stach, B. (1985). Auditory brainstem response testing strategies. In J. T. Jacobson (Ed.), *The auditory brainstem response* (pp. 371–388). San Diego, CA: College-Hill Press.

Jewett, D. (1969). Averaged volume-conducted potentials to auditory stimuli in the cat. *Physiologist, 12,* 262.

Jewett, D. (1970). Volume-conducted potentials to auditory stimuli as detected by averaging in the cat. *Electroencephalography and Clinical Neurophysiology, 28,* 609–618.

Jewett, D., Romano, M., & Williston, J. (1970). Human auditory evoked potentials: Possible brainstem components detected on the scalp. *Science, 167,* 1517–1518.

Jewett, D., & Williston, J. (1971). Auditory evoked far fields averaged from the scalp of humans. *Brain, 94,* 681–696.

Jones, T. A., Stockard, J. J., & Weidner, W. J. (1980). The effects of temperature and acute alcohol intoxication on brain stem auditory evoked potentials in the cat. *Electroencephalography and Clinical Neurophysiology, 49,* 23–30.

Kaga, K., Nakamura, M., Shinogami, M., Tsuzuku, T., Yamada, K., & Shindo, M. (1996). Auditory nerve disease of both ears revealed by auditory brainstem responses, electrocochleography and otoacoustic emissions. *Scandinavian Audiology, 25,* 233–238.

Katbamna, B., Metz, D. A., Bennett, S. L., & Dokler, P. A. (1996). Effects of electrode montage on the spectral composition of the infant auditory brainstem response. *Journal of the American Academy of Audiology, 7,* 269–273.

Kemp, D. T., Ryan, S., & Bray, P. (1990). A guide to the effective use of otoacoustic emissions. *Ear and Hearing, 11,* 93–105.

Kevanishvili, Z., & Aphonchenko, V. (1981). Click polarity inversion effects upon the human auditory evoked potential. *Scandinavian Audiology, 10,* 141–147.

Kileny, P. (1981). The frequency specificity of tone-pip evoked auditory brain stem responses. *Ear and Hearing, 2,* 270–275.

Killion, M. C. (1984). New insert earphones for audiometry. *Hearing Instruments, 35,* 28, 46.

Killion, M., Wilber, L., & Gudmundsen, G. (1985). Insert earphones for more interaural attenuation. *Hearing Instruments, 36,* 34–36.

Kjaer, M. (1979). Differences of latencies and amplitudes of brain stem evoked potentials in subgroups of a normal material. *Acta Neurologica Scandinavia, 59,* 72–79.

Klein, A. J. (1983). Properties of the brain-stem response slow-wave component. *Archives of Otolaryngology, 109,* 6–12.

Kodera, K., Yamane, H., Yamada, O., & Suzuki, J. (1977). Brain stem response audiometry at speech frequencies. *Audiology, 16,* 469–479.

Kraus, N., & McGee, T. (1992). Electrophysiology of the human auditory system. In A. N. Popper & R. R. Fay (Eds.), *The mammalian auditory pathway: Neurophysiology.* New York: Springer-Verlag.

Kraus, N., McGee, T., Carrell, T. D., & Sharma, A. (1995). Neurophysiologic bases of speech discrimination. *Ear and Hearing, 16,* 19–37.

Kraus, N., Özdamar, Ö., Heydemann, P. T., Stein, L., & Reed, N. (1984). Auditory brain-stem responses in hydrocephalic patients. *Electroencephalography and Clinical Neurophysiology, 59,* 310–317.

Kraus, N., Özdamar, Ö., Stein, L., & Reed, N. (1984). Absent auditory brain stem response: Peripheral hearing loss or brain stem dysfunction? *Laryngoscope, 94,* 400–406.

Lafreniere, O., Smurzynski, J., Jung, M. D., Leonard, G., & Kim D. O. (1993). Otoacoustic emissions in full-term newborns at risk for hearing loss. *Laryngoscope, 103,* 1334–1341.

Lasky, R. E., Shi, Y., & Hecox, K. E. (1993). Binaural maximum length sequence auditory-evoked brain-stem responses in human adults. *Journal of the Acoustical Society of America, 93,* 2077–2087.

Lazor, J., & Melnick, W. (1984). A survey of current clinical procedures in use by audiologists to measure auditory brainstem responses. In A. Starr, C. Rosenberg, M. Don, & H. Davis (Eds.), *Sensory evoked potentials: I. An international conference on standards for auditory brain stem response (ABR) testing.* Milan, Italy: Edizion Techniche Cura del Centro Richerche Stud. Amplifon Ellectrofisiologia.

Lettrem, I., & Laukli, E. (1995). Analog and digital filtering of ABR: Ipsi- and contralateral derivations. *Ear and Hearing, 16,* 508–514.

Lina-Grande, G., Collet, L., & Morgon, A. (1994). Auditory-evoked brainstem responses elicited by maximum-length sequences in normal and sensorineural ears. *Audiology, 33,* 218–236.

Lins, O. G., & Picton, T. W. (1995). Auditory steady-state responses to multiple simultaneous stimuli. *Electroencephalography and Clinical Neurophysiology, 96,* 420–432.

Lins, O. G., Picton, T. W., Boucher, B. L., Dureiux-Smith, A., Champagne, S. C., Moran, L. M., Perez-Abalo, M. C., Martin, V., & Savio, G. (1996). Frequency-specific audiometry using steady-state responses. *Ear and Hearing, 17,* 81–96.

Martin, M., & Moore, E. (1977). Scalp distribution of early (0 to 10 msec) auditory evoked responses. *Archives of Otolaryngology, 103,* 326–328.

Mason, S. M. (1984). On-line computer scoring of the auditory brainstem response for estimation of hearing threshold. *Audiology, 23,* 277–296.

Maurer, K. (1985). Uncertainties of topodiagnosis of auditory nerve and brainstem auditory evoked potentials due to rarefaction and condensation stimuli. *Electroencephalography and Clinical Neurophysiology, 62,* 135–140.

Maurer, K., Schafer, E., & Leitner, H. (1980). The effect of varying stimulus polarity (rarefaction vs. condensation) on early auditory evoked potentials (EAEPs). *Electroencephalography and Clinical Neurophysiology, 50,* 332–334.

McGee, T. J., & Clemis, J. D. (1982). Effects of conductive hearing loss on auditory brainstem response. *Annals of Otology, Rhinology and Laryngology, 91,* 304–309.

McPherson, D. L. (1996). *Late potentials of the auditory system.* San Diego, CA: Singular Publishing Group.

McPherson, D. L., & Starr, A. (1993). Binaural interaction in auditory evoked potentials: Brainstem, middle- and long-latency components. *Hearing Research, 66,* 91–98.

Mendelson, T., Salamy, A., Lenoir, M., & McKean, C. (1979). Brain stem evoked potential findings in children with otitis media. *Archives of Otolaryngology, 105,* 17–20.

Michalewski, H. J., Thompson, L. W., Patterson, J. V., Bowman, T. E., & Litzelman, D. (1980). Sex differences in the amplitudes and latencies of the human auditory brain stem potential. *Electroencephalography and Clinical Neurophysiology, 48,* 351–356.

Mizrahi, E. M., Maulsby, R. L., & Frost, J. D., Jr. (1983). Improved Wave V resolution by dual-channel brain stem auditory evoked potential recording. *Electroencephalography and Clinical Neurophysiology, 55,* 105–107.

Mjøen, S., Nordby, H. K., & Torvik, A. (1983). Auditory evoked brainstem response (ABR) in coma due to severe head trauma. *Acta Otolaryngologica (Stockholm), 85,* 131–138.

Mokotoff, B., Schulman-Galambos, C., & Galambos, R. (1977). Brain stem auditory evoked responses in children. *Archives of Otolaryngology, 103,* 38–43.

Møller, A. R. (1994). Neural generators of auditory evoked potentials. In J. T. Jacobson (Ed.), *Principles and applications in auditory evoked potentials.* Boston: Allyn & Bacon.

Møller, A. R., & Jannetta, P. J. (1981). Compound action potentials recorded intracranially from the auditory nerve in man. *Experimental Neurology, 74,* 862–874.

Møller, A. R., & Jannetta, P. J. (1982). Auditory evoked potentials recorded intracranially from the brainstem in man. *Experimental Neurology, 78,* 144–157.

Møller, A. R., Jannetta, P. J., & Sekhar, L. N. (1988). Contributions from the auditory nerve to the brainstem auditory evoked potentials (BAEPs): Results of intracranial recording in man. *Electroencephalography and Clinical Neurophysiology, 71,* 198–211.

Møller, K., & Blegvad, B. (1976). Brain stem responses in patients with sensorineural hearing loss. *Scandinavian Audiology, 5,* 115–127.

Møller, M. B., & Møller, A. R. (1983). Brainstem auditory evoked potentials in patients with cerebellopontine angle tumors. *Annals of Otology, Rhinology and Laryngology, 92,* 645–650.

Moore, J. K. (1987). The human auditory brain stem as a generator of auditory evoked potentials. *Hearing Research, 29,* 33–44.

Moore, J. K., Ponton, C. W., Eggermont, J. J., Wu, B. J., & Huang, J. Q. (1996). Perinatal maturation of the auditory brain stem response: Changes in path length and conduction velocity. *Ear and Hearing, 17,* 411–418.

Musiek, F. E., Gollegly, K. M., Kibbe, K. S., & Verkest, S. B. (1988). Current concepts on the use of ABR and auditory psychophysical tests in evaluation of brain stem lesions. *American Journal of Otology, 9* (Suppl.), 25–35.

Musiek, F. E., Johnson, G. D., Gollegly, K. M., Josey, A. F., & Glasscock, M. E. (1989). The auditory brain stem response interaural latency difference (ILD) in patients with brain stem lesions. *Ear and Hearing, 10,* 131–134.

Musiek, F. E., Josey, A. F., & Glasscock, M. E., III. (1986). Auditory brain-stem response in patients with acoustic neuromas. *Archives of Otolaryngology, 112,* 186–189.

Musiek, F. E., Kibbe, K., Rackliffe, L., & Weider, D. J. (1984). The auditory brain stem response I-V amplitude ratio in normal, cochlear, and retrocochlear ears. *Ear and Hearing, 5,* 52–55.

Musiek, F. E., Kibbe-Michal, K., Geurkink, N. A., & Josey, A. F. (1986). ABR results in patients with posterior fossa tumors and normal pure-tone hearing. *Otolaryngology— Head and Neck Surgery, 94,* 568–573.

Musiek, F. E., & Lee, W. W. (1995). The auditory brain stem response in patients with brain stem or cochlear pathology. *Ear and Hearing, 16,* 631–636.

Naessens, B., Gordts, F., Clement, P. A., & Buisseret, T. (1996). Re-evaluation of the ABR in the diagnosis of CPA tumors in the MRI-era. *Acta Oto-Rhino-Laryngologica Belgica, 50,* 99–102.

Newton, V. E., & Barratt, H. J. (1983). An evaluation of the use of the auditory brainstem electric response test in paediatric audiological assessment. *International Journal of Pediatric Otorhinolaryngology, 5,* 139–149.

Nodar, R., Hahn, J., & Levine, H. (1980). Brain stem auditory evoked potentials in determining site of lesion of brain stem gliomas in children. *Laryngoscope, 90,* 258–266.

Nodar, R., & Kinney, S. (1980). The contralateral effects of large tumors on brain stem auditory evoked potentials. *Laryngoscope, 90,* 1762–1768.

Norton, S. J., & Widen, J. E. (1990). Evoked otoacoustic emissions in normal-hearing infants and children: Emerging data and issues. *Ear and Hearing, 11,* 121–127.

Orlando, M. S., & Folsom, R. C. (1995). The effects of reversing the polarity of frequency-limited single-cycle stimuli on the human auditory brain stem response. *Ear and Hearing, 16,* 311–320.

Ottaviani, F., Almadori, G., Calderazzo, A. B., Frenguelli, A., & Paludetti, G. (1986). Auditory brain-stem (ABRs) and middle latency auditory responses (MLRs) in the prognosis of severely head-injured patients. *Electroencephalography and Clinical Neurophysiology, 65,* 196–202.

Otto, W. C., & McCandless, G. A. (1982). Aging and the auditory brain stem response. *Audiology, 21,* 466–473.

Özdamar, Ö., & Delgado, R. E. (1996). Measurement of signal and noise characteristics in ongoing auditory brainstem response averaging. *Annals of Biomedical Engineering, 24,* 702–715.

Özdamar, Ö., Delgado, R. E., Eilers, R. E., & Urbano, R. C. (1994). Automated electrophysiologic hearing testing using a threshold-seeking algorithm. *Journal of the American Academy of Audiology, 5,* 77–88.

Özdamar, Ö., & Kraus, N. (1983). Auditory brainstem response in infants recovering from meningitis: Neurologic assessment. *Archives of Neurology, 40,* 499–502.

Özdamar, Ö., & Stein, L. (1981). Auditory brain stem response (ABR) in unilateral hearing loss. *Laryngoscope, 91,* 565–574.

Paludetti, G., Maurizi, M., & Ottaviani, F. (1983). Effects of stimulus repetition rate on the auditory brain stem responses (ABR). *American Journal of Otology, 4,* 226–234.

Parker, D. J., & Thornton, A. R. D. (1978a). Frequency specific components of the cochlear nerve and brainstem evoked responses of the human auditory system. *Scandinavian Audiology, 7,* 53–60.

Parker, D. J., & Thornton, A. R. D. (1978b). The validity of the derived cochlear nerve and brainstem evoked responses of the human auditory system. *Scandinavian Audiology, 7,* 45–52.

Picton, T. W. (1978). The strategy of evoked potential audiometry. In S. E. Gerber & G. T. Mencher (Eds.), *Early diagnosis of hearing loss* (pp. 279–307). New York: Grune & Stratton.

Picton, T. W., Champagne, S. C., & Kellett, A. J. C. (1992). Human auditory evoked potentials recorded using maximum length sequences. *Electroencephalography and Clinical Neurophysiology, 84,* 90–100.

Picton, T. W., & Hillyard, S. A. (1974). Human auditory evoked potentials: II. Effects of attention. *Electroencephalography and Clinical Neurophysiology, 36,* 191–199.

Picton, T. W., Hillyard, S. A., Krausz, H. I., & Galambos, R. (1974). Human auditory evoked potentials: I. Evaluation of components. *Electroencephalography and Clinical Neurophysiology, 36,* 179–190.

Picton, T. W., Ouellette, J., Hamel, G., & Smith, A. (1979). Brainstem evoked potentials to tone pips in notched noise. *Journal of Otolaryngology, 8,* 289–314.

Picton, T. W., Skinner, C. R., Champagne, S. C., Kellet, A. J. C., & Maiste, A. C. (1987). Potentials evoked by the sinusoidal modulation of the amplitude or frequency of a tone. *Journal of the Acoustical Society of America, 82,* 165–178.

Picton, T. W., Woods, D. L., Baribeau-Braun, J., & Healey, T. M. G. (1977). Evoked potential audiometry. *Journal of Otolaryngology, 6,* 90–119.

Pikus, A. T. (1995). Pediatric audiologic profile in type 1 and type 2 neurofibromatosis. *Journal of the American Academy of Audiology, 6,* 54–62.

Polyakov, A., & Pratt, H. (1995). The effect of broad-band noise on the binaural interaction components of human auditory brainstem-evoked potentials. *Audiology, 34,* 36–46.

Pool, K. D., & Finitzo, T. (1989). Evaluation of a computer-automated program for clinical assessment of the auditory brain stem response. *Ear and Hearing, 10,* 304–310.

Pratt, H., & Bleich, N. (1982). Auditory brain stem potentials evoked by clicks in notch-filtered masking noise. *Electroencephalography and Clinical Neurophysiology, 53,* 417–426.

Pratt, H., Bleich, N., & Martin, W. H. (1985). Three-channel Lissajous' trajectory of human auditory brain-stem evoked potentials: I. Normative measures. *Electroencephalography and Clinical Neurophysiology, 61,* 530–538.

Pratt, H., & Sohmer, H. (1976). Intensity and rate functions of cochlear and brain stem evoked responses to click stimuli in man. *Archives of Oto-Rhino-Laryngology (Berlin), 212,* 85–92.

Pratt, H., & Sohmer, H. (1978). Comparison of hearing threshold determined by auditory pathway electrical responses and by behavioral responses. *Audiology, 17,* 285–292.

Rance, G., Rickards, F. W., Cohen, L. T., De Vidi, S., & Clark, G. M. (1995). The automated prediction of hearing thresholds in sleeping subjects using auditory steady-state evoked potentials. *Ear and Hearing, 16,* 499–507.

Rickards, F. W., & Clark, G. M. (1984). Steady state evoked potentials to amplitude-modulated tones. In C. Barber, & R. H. Nodar, (Eds.), *Evoked potentials II* (pp. 163–168). Boston, MA: Butterworth.

Roberson, J., Senne, A., Brackmann, D., Hitselberger, W. E., & Saunders, J. (1996). Direct cochlear nerve action potentials as an aid to hearing preservation in middle fossa acoustic neuroma resection. *American Journal of Otology, 17,* 653–657.

Robinson, K., & Rudge, P. (1977). Abnormalities of auditory evoked potentials in patients with multiple sclerosis. *Brain, 100,* 19–40.

Rosenhamer, H. (1977). Observations on electric brain-stem responses in retrocochlear hearing loss. *Scandinavian Audiology, 6,* 179–196.

Rosenhamer, H., Lindstrom, B., & Lundborg, T. (1978). On the use of click evoked electric brainstem responses in audiological diagnosis: I. The variability of the normal response. *Scandinavian Audiology, 7,* 193–205.

Rosenhamer, H., Lindstrom, B., & Lundborg, T. (1981). On the use of click evoked electric brainstem responses in audiological diagnosis: IV. Differences in cochlear hearing. *Scandinavian Audiology, 10,* 67–73.

Rowe, M. J., III. (1978). Normal variability of the brain-stem auditory evoked response in young and old adult subjects. *Electroencephalography and Clinical Neurophysiology, 44,* 459–470.

Rubel, E. W., & Ryals, B. M. (1983). Development of the place principle: Acoustic trauma. *Science, 219,* 512–514.

Ruben, R. J., Bordley, J. E., & Lieberman, A. T. (1961). Cochlear potentials in man. *Laryngoscope, 71,* 1141–1164.

Ryan, A. F., Woolf, N. K., & Sharp, F. R. (1982). Functional ontogeny in the central auditory pathway of the mongolian gerbil: A deoxyglucose study. *Experimental Brain Research, 47,* 428–436.

Salamy, A., McKean, C., & Buda, F. (1975). Maturational changes in auditory transmission as reflected in human brain stem potentials. *Brain Research, 96,* 361–366.

Sanchez, R., Riquenes, A., & Perez-Abalo, M. (1995). Automatic detection of auditory brainstem responses using feature vectors. *International Journal of Bio-Medical Computing, 39,* 287–297.

Sanders, R. A., Duncan, P. G., & McCullough, D. W. (1979). Clinical experience with brain stem audiometry performed under general anesthesia. *Journal of Otolaryngology, 8,* 31–38.

Sanders, R., Smirga, D., McCullough, D., & Duncan, P. (1981). Auditory brain stem response in patients with global cerebral insults. *Journal of Otolaryngology, 10,* 34–41.

Scherg, M., & von Cramon, D. (1985). A new interpretation of the generators of BAEP waves I-V: Results of a spatial-temporal dipole. *Electroencephalography and Clinical Neurophysiology, 62,* 290–299.

Schoonhoven, R. (1992). Dependence of auditory brainstem response on click polarity and high-frequency sensorineural hearing loss. *Audiology, 31,* 72–86.

Schulman-Galambos, C., & Galambos, R. (1975). Brain stem auditory-evoked responses in premature infants. *Journal of Speech and Hearing Research, 18,* 456–465.

Schulman-Galambos, C., & Galambos, R. (1979). Brain stem evoked response audiometry in newborn hearing screening. *Archives of Otolaryngology, 105,* 86–90.

Schwartz, D. M., Larson, V., & DeChicchis, A. R. (1985). Spectral characteristics of air and bone transducers used to record the auditory brainstem response. *Ear and Hearing, 6,* 274–277.

Seales, D., Rossiter, V., & Weinstein, M. (1979). Brainstem auditory evoked responses in patients comatose as a result of blunt head trauma. *Journal of Trauma, 19,* 347–353.

Sells, J. P., & Hurley, R. M. (1994). Acoustic neuroma in an adolescent without neurofibromatosis: Case study. *Journal of the American Academy of Audiology, 5,* 349–354.

Selters, W., & Brackmann, D. (1977). Acoustic tumor detection with brain stem electric response audiometry. *Archives of Otolaryngology, 103,* 181–187.

Selters, W., & Brackmann, D. (1979). Brainstem electric response audiometry in acoustic tumor detection. In W. F. House & C. M. Luetje (Eds.), *Acoustic tumors* (pp. 225–235). Baltimore: University Park Press.

Shanon, E., Gold, S., & Himmelfarb, M. (1981). Auditory brain stem responses in cerebellopontine angle tumors. *Laryngoscope, 91,* 254–259.

Sidman, J. D., Carrasco, V. N., Whaley, R. A., & Pillsbury, H. C., III. (1989). Gadolinium: The new gold standard for diagnosing cerebellopontine angle tumors. *Archives of Otolaryngology—Head and Neck Surgery, 115,* 1244–1247.

Sininger, Y. S. (1992). Establishing clinical norms for auditory brainstem response. *American Journal of Audiology, 1,* 16–18.

Sininger, Y. S. (1993). Auditory brain stem response for objective measures of hearing. *Ear and Hearing, 14,* 23–30.

Sininger, Y. S. (1995). Filtering and spectral characteristics of average auditory brain-stem response and background noise in infants. *Journal of the Acoustical Society of America, 98,* 2048–2055.

Sininger, Y. S., & Abdala, C. (1998). Physiologic assessment of hearing. In A. K. Lalwani, & K. M. Grundfast, (Eds.), *Pediatric otology and neurotology* (pp. 127–154). Philadelphia, PA: Lippincott-Raven.

Sininger, Y. S., Abdala, C., & Cone-Wesson, B. (1997). Auditory threshold sensitivity of the human neonate as measured by the auditory brainstem response. *Hearing Research, 104,* 27–38.

Sininger, Y. S., Hood, L. J., Starr, A., Berlin, C. I., & Picton, T. W. (1995). Hearing loss due to auditory neuropathy. *Audiology Today, 7,* 10–13.

Sininger, Y. S., & Masuda, A. (1990). Effect of click polarity on ABR threshold. *Ear and Hearing, 11,* 206–209.

Smith, L. E., & Simmons, F. B. (1982). Accuracy of auditory brainstem evoked response with hearing level unknown. *Annals of Otology, Rhinology and Laryngology, 91,* 266–267.

Sohmer, H., & Feinmesser, M. (1967). Cochlear action potentials recorded from the external ear in man. *Annals of Otology, Rhinology and Laryngology, 76,* 427–435.

Sohmer, H., Feinmesser, M., & Szabo, G. (1974). Sources of electrocochleographic responses as studied in patients with brain damage. *Electroencephalography and Clinical Neurophysiology, 37,* 663–669.

Sostarich, M. E., Ferraro, J. A., & Karlsen, E. A. (1993). Prolonged I–III interwave interval in cerebellar astrocytoma. *Journal of the American Academy of Audiology, 4,* 269–271.

Spivak, L. (1993). Spectral composition of infant auditory brainstem responses: Implications for filtering. *Audiology, 32,* 185–194.

Squires, K., Chu, N., & Starr, A. (1978). Acute effect of alcohol on auditory brainstem potentials in man. *Science, 201,* 174–176.

Stach, B. A., & Delgado-Vilches, G. (1993). Sudden hearing loss in multiple sclerosis: Case report. *Journal of the American Academy of Audiology, 4,* 370–375.

Stach, B. A., Wolf, S. J., & Bland, L. (1995). Otoacoustic emissions as a cross-check in pediatric hearing assessment: Case report. *Journal of the American Academy of Audiology, 4,* 392–398.

Stack, J. P., Antoun, N. M., Jenkins, J. P. R., Metcalfe, R., & Isherwood, I. (1988). Gadolinium-DTPA as a contrast agent in magnetic resonance imaging of the brain. *Neuroradiology, 30,* 145–154.

Stanton, S. G., & Cashman, M. Z. (1996). Auditory brainstem response. A comparison of different interpretation strategies for detection of cerebellopontine angle tumors. *Scandinavian Audiology, 25,* 109–120.

Stapells, D. R., Gravel, J. S., & Martin, B. A. (1995). Thresholds for auditory brain stem responses to tones in notched noise from infants and young children with normal hearing and sensorineural hearing loss. *Ear and Hearing, 16,* 361–371.

Stapells, D. R., Linden, D., Suffield, J. B., Hamel, G., & Picton, T. W. (1984). Human auditory steady state potentials. *Ear and Hearing, 5,* 105–113.

Stapells, D. R., & Picton, T. W. (1981). Technical aspects of brainstem evoked audiometry using tones. *Ear and Hearing, 2,* 20–29.

Stapells, D. R., Picton, T. W., Durieux-Smith, A., Edwards, C. G., & Moran, L. M. (1990). Thresholds for short-latency auditory evoked potentials to tones in notched noise in normal-hearing and hearing-impaired subjects. *Audiology, 29,* 262–274.

Stapells, D. R., Picton, T. W., Perez-Abalo, M., Read, D., & Smith, A. (1985). Frequency specific evoked potential audiometry. In J. T. Jacobson (Ed.), *The auditory brainstem response* (pp. 145–177). San Diego, CA: College-Hill Press.

Stapells, D. R., Picton, T. W., & Smith, A. D. (1982). Normal hearing thresholds for clicks. *Journal of the Acoustical Society of America, 72,* 74–79.

Starr, A. (1977). Clinical relevance of brain stem auditory evoked potentials in brain stem disorders in man. Auditory evoked potentials in man. Psychopharmacology correlates of EPs. In J. E. Desmedt (Ed.), *Programs in clinical neurophysiology* (Vol. 2, pp. 45–57). Basel, Switzerland: Karger.

Starr, A., & Achor, L. J. (1975). Auditory brain stem responses in neurological disease. *Archives of Neurology, 32,* 761–768.

Starr, A., Amlie, R. N., Martin, W. H., & Sanders, S. (1977). Development of auditory function in newborn infants revealed by auditory brainstem potentials. *Pediatrics, 60,* 831–839.

Starr, A., & Hamilton, A. (1976). Correlation between confirmed sites of neurological lesions and abnormalities of far-field auditory brainstem responses. *Electroencephalography and Clinical Neurophysiology, 41,* 595–608.

Starr, A., McPherson, D., Patterson, J., Don, M., Luxford, W., Shannon, R., Sininger, Y., Tonokawa, L., & Waring, M. (1991). Absence of both auditory evoked potentials and auditory percepts dependent on timing cues. *Brain, 114,* 1157–1180.

Starr, A., Picton, T. W., Sininger, Y. S., Hood, L. J., & Berlin, C. I. (1996). Auditory neuropathy. *Brain, 119,* 741–753.

Stein, L. K., Kraus, N., Özdamar, Ö., Cartee, C., Jabaley, T., Jeantet, C., & Reed, N. (1987). Hearing loss in an institutionalized mentally retarded population: Identification by auditory brainstem response. *Archives of Otolaryngology—Head and Neck Surgery, 113,* 32–35.

Stein, L. K., Özdamar, Ö., & Schnabel, M. (1981). Auditory brainstem responses (ABR) with suspected deaf-blind children. *Ear and Hearing, 2,* 30–40.

Stein, L., Tremblay, K., Pasternak, J., Banerjee, S., Lindemann, K., & Kraus, N. (1996). Brainstem abnormalities in neonates with normal otoacoustic emissions. *Seminars in Hearing, 17,* 197–213.

Stockard, J. J., & Rossiter, V. (1977). Clinical and pathological correlates of brain stem auditory response abnormalities. *Neurology, 27,* 316–325.

Stockard, J. J., Rossiter, V. S., Jones, T. A., & Sharbrough, F. W. (1977). Effects of centrally acting drugs on brainstem auditory responses. *Electroencephalography and Clinical Neurophysiology, 43,* 550–551.

Stockard, J. J., Sharbrough, F. W., & Tinker, J. A. (1978). Effects of hypothermia on the human brainstem response. *Annals of Neurology, 3,* 368–370.

Stockard, J. J., & Stockard, J. E. (1981). Clinical applications: Recording and analyzing. In E. Moore (Ed.), *Electrocochleography and brainstem electric audiometry* (pp. 255–286). New York: Grune and Stratton.

Stockard, J. J., Stockard, J. E., & Sharbrough, F. W. (1978). Nonpathologic factors influencing brainstem auditory evoked potentials. *American Journal of EEG Technicians, 18,* 177–209.

Stockard, J. J., Stockard, J. E., & Sharbrough, F. W. (1980). Brainstem auditory evoked potentials in neurology: Methodology, interpretation, clinical application. In M. J. Aminoff (Ed.), *Electrodiagnosis in clinical neurology* (pp. 370–413). New York: Churchill Livingstone.

Stockard, J. J., Stockard, J. E., Westmoreland, B., & Corfits, J. (1979). Brainstem auditory-evoked responses: Normal variation as a function of stimulus and subject characteristics. *Archives of Neurology, 36,* 823–831.

Stuart, A., & Yang, E. Y. (1994). Effect of high-pass filtering on the neonatal auditory brainstem response to air- and bone-conducted clicks. *Journal of Speech and Hearing Research, 37,* 475–479.

Stuart, A., Yang, E. Y., & Stenstrom, R. (1990). Effect of temporal area bone vibrator placement on auditory brain stem response in newborn infants. *Ear and Hearing, 11,* 363–369.

Student, M., & Sohmer, H. (1978). Evidence from auditory nerve and brainstem evoked responses for an organic brain lesion in children with autistic traits. *Journal of Autism and Childhood Schizophrenia, 8,* 13–20.

Stypulkowski, P. H., & Staller, S. J. (1987). Clinical evaluation of a new ECoG recording electrode. *Ear and Hearing, 8,* 304–310.

Tanaka, H., Komatsuzaki, A., & Hentona, H. (1996). Usefulness of auditory brainstem responses at high stimulus rates in the diagnosis of acoustic neuroma. *Journal of Oto-Rhino-Laryngology, 58,* 224–228.

Teas, D. C., Eldredge, D. H., & Davis, H. (1962). Cochlear responses to acoustic transients: An interpretation of whole-nerve action potentials. *Journal of the Acoustical Society of America, 34,* 1438–1459.

Telian, S. A., & Kileny, P. R. (1988). Pitfalls in neurotologic diagnosis. *Ear and Hearing, 9,* 86–91.

Telian, S. A., & Kileny, P. R. (1989). Usefulness of 1000 Hz tone-burst-evoked responses in the diagnosis of acoustic neuroma. *Otolaryngology—Head and Neck Surgery, 101,* 466–471.

Terkildsen, K., Huis in't Veld, F., & Osterhammel, P. (1977). Auditory brain stem responses in the diagnosis of cerebellopontine angle tumors. *Scandinavian Audiology, 6,* 43–47.

Terkildsen, K., Osterhammel, P., & Huis in't Veld, F. (1975). Far-field electrocochleography: Frequency specificity of the response. *Scandinavian Audiology, 4,* 167–172.

Thomason, J. E.-M., Smyth, V., & Murdoch, B. E. (1993). Acoustic neuroma and non-tumor retrocochlear patients: Audiological features. *Scandinavian Audiology, 22,* 19–23.

Thomsen, J., Terkildsen, K., & Osterhammel, P. (1978). Auditory brain stem responses in patients with acoustic neuromas. *Scandinavian Audiology, 7,* 179–183.

Thornton, A. R. D. (1980). Audiological and neurological applications of cochlear and brainstem evoked response. *Hearing Instruments, 31,* 14–21.

Thornton, A. R., Mendel, M. I., & Anderson, C. V. (1977). Effects of stimulus frequency and intensity on the middle components of the averaged auditory electroencephalic response. *Journal of Speech and Hearing Research, 20,* 81–94.

Thornton, A. R., & Slaven, A. (1993). Auditory brainstem responses recorded at fast stimulation rates using maximum length sequences. *British Journal of Audiology, 27,* 205–210.

Tucci, D. L., Telian, S. A., Kileny, P. R., Hoff, J. T., & Kemick, J. L. (1994). Stability of hearing preservation following acoustic neuroma surgery. *American Journal of Otology, 15,* 183–188.

Valente, M., Peterein, J., Goebel, J., & Neely, J. G. (1995). Four cases of acoustic neuromas with normal hearing. *Journal of the American Academy of Audiology, 6,* 203–210.

Van Campen, L. E., Sammeth, C. A., Hall, J. W., III, & Peek, B. F. (1992). Comparison of Etymotic insert and TDH supra-aural earphones in auditory brainstem response measurement. *Journal of the American Academy of Audiology, 3,* 315–323.

van Olphen, A. F., Rodenburg, M., & Verwey, C. (1979). Influence of stimulus repetition rate on brain-stem-evoked responses in man. *Audiology, 18,* 388–394.

Ventry, I., Chaiklin, J., & Boyle, W. I. (1962). Collapse of the ear canal during audiometry. *Archives of Otolaryngology, 75,* 422–423.

Virtaniemi, J., Laakso, M., Karja, J., Nuutinen, J., & Karjalainen, S. (1993). Auditory brainstem latencies in type I (insulin-dependent) diabetic patients. *American Journal of Otolaryngology, 14,* 413–418.

Watson, D. R. (1996). The effects of cochlear hearing loss, age and sex on the auditory brainstem response. *Audiology, 35,* 246–258.

Wazen, J. J. (1994). Intraoperative monitoring of auditory function: Experimental observations and new applications. *Laryngoscope, 104,* 446–455.

Weber, B. A. (1982). Comparison of auditory brain stem response latency norms for premature infants. *Ear and Hearing, 3,* 257–262.

Weber, B. A., & Roush, P. A. (1993). Application of maximum length sequence analysis to auditory brainstem response testing of premature newborns. *Journal of the American Academy of Audiology, 4,* 157–162.

Weber, B. A., Seitz, M. R., & McCutcheon, M. J. (1981). Quantifying click stimuli in auditory brainstem response audiometry. *Ear and Hearing, 2,* 15–19.

Webster, D. B. (1995). *Neuroscience of communication.* San Diego, CA: Singular Publishing Group.

Wever, E. G., & Bray, C. W. (1930). Auditory nerve impulses. *Science, 71,* 215.

Widen, J. E. (1997). Evoked otoacoustic emissions in evaluating children. In M. S. Robinette & T. J. Glattke (Eds.), *Otoacoustic emissions: Clinical applications.* New York: Thieme.

Worthington, D. W., & Peters, J. F. (1980). Quantifiable hearing and no ABR: Paradox or error? *Ear and Hearing, 1,* 281–285.

Yamada, O., Kodera, K., & Yagi, T. (1979). Cochlear processes affecting Wave V latency of the auditory evoked brain stem response. *Scandinavian Audiology, 8,* 67–70.

Yang, E. Y., Rupert, A. L., & Moushegian, G. (1987). A developmental study of bone conduction auditory brain stem responses in infants. *Ear and Hearing, 8,* 244–251.

Yang, E., Stuart, A., Mencher, G. T., Mencher, L. S., & Vincer, M. J. (1993). Auditory brain stem responses to air- and bone-conducted clicks in the audiological assessment of at-risk infants. *Ear and Hearing, 14,* 175–182:

Yang, E. Y., Stuart, A., Stenstrom, R., & Green, W. B. (1993). Test-retest variability of the auditory brainstem response to bone-conducted clicks in newborn infants. *Audiology, 32,* 89–94.

Yellin, M. W., Jerger, J., & Fifer, R. C. (1989). Norms for disproportionate loss in speech intelligibility. *Ear and Hearing, 10,* 231–234.

Zimmerman, M. C., Morgan, D. E., & Dubno, J. R. (1987). Auditory brain stem evoked response characteristics in developing infants. *Annals of Otology, Rhinology and Laryngology, 96,* 291–299.

I

Index